THE
FastLife

THE
FastLife

Lose Weight, Stay Healthy, and Live Longer with
the Simple Secrets of Intermittent Fasting and
High-Intensity Training

Dr. Michael Mosley
and Mimi Spencer
with Peta Bee

ATRIA PAPERBACK
New York   London   Toronto   Sydney   New Delhi

ATRIA PAPERBACK

An Imprint of Simon & Schuster, Inc.
1230 Avenue of the Americas
New York, NY 10020

First Atria Paperback edition September 2015

ATRIA PAPERBACK and colophon are trademarks of
Simon & Schuster, Inc.

For information about special discounts for bulk purchases, please
contact Simon & Schuster Special Sales at 1-866-506-1949 or business@
simonandschuster.com.

The Simon & Schuster Speakers Bureau can bring authors to your live
event. For more information or to book an event, contact the Simon &
Schuster Speakers Bureau at 1-866-248-3049 or visit our website at
www.simonspeakers.com.

Manufactured in the United States of America

10   9   8   7   6   5   4   3   2

Library of Congress Cataloging-in-Publication Data

Mosley, Michael.
    The FastLife : lose weight, stay healthy, and live longer with the simple
secrets of intermittent fasting and high-intensity training / Dr. Michael
Mosley, Mimi Spencer.—First Atria Paperback edition.
        pages cm
Summary: "Finally in one comprehensive volume—Dr. Michael Mosley's
#1 New York Times bestseller The FastDiet and his results-driven high-
intensity training program FastExercise combine for the ultimate one-stop
health and wellness guide that helps you reinvent your body the Fast
way!"—Provided by publisher.
    Includes bibliographical references and index.
    1. Reducing diets—Recipes. 2. Intermittent fasting. 3. Exercise. I.
Spencer, Mimi, 1967- II. Title.
    RM222.2.M653 2015
    613.2'5—dc23
                                        2015026606

ISBN 978-1-5011-2798-4
ISBN 978-1-5011-2867-7 (ebook)

For my wife, Clare, and children, Alex, Jack, Daniel,
and Kate, who make living longer worthwhile.

—M.M.

For Ned, Lily May, and Paul—my Brighton rock. And for
my parents, who have always known that food is love.

—M.S.

Contents

Contents

Foreword

On my first day as a medical student at the Royal Free Hospital School of Medicine, part of the University of London, I sat down with a hundred others in a huge lecture hall to be greeted by the dean. He talked for over an hour about how lucky we were to be there, our potentially glorious future, and the importance of being kind to patients.

There are, specifically, two things he said that I still remember very clearly. The first was that, based on previous experience, four of us in that room would marry each other. He was right; I met my future wife that day.

The other thing he said that really struck me was that while we would learn an enormous amount over the first five years of our training, within ten years of graduating much of what we had learned would be out-of-date.

Medicine and nutrition are disciplines where the "truth" is constantly changing. New studies come along that sometimes reinforce and sometimes undermine established wisdom. Unless you keep up with the latest research, you are doomed to cling to outdated ideas.

It has been two years since we wrote the first edition of *The FastDiet*, and over that period a great deal has changed, so we decided it was time to update the book.

There have been a number of new studies on intermittent fasting and high-intensity training that I wanted to include.

There are also important health areas that we didn't feel ready to include in the original book, but that we have been frequently asked about, including research into the effects of intermittent fasting on inflammatory diseases such as asthma, eczema, and psoriasis.

We have included an expanded section on exercise, as it is clear that combining exercise with intermittent fasting is likely to lead to greater improvements. There is also an interesting new study that has looked at the effects of combining intermittent fasting with a novel form of exercise, high-intensity training.

Then there's the all-important question of what you should eat on your fasting days. Mimi has created a whole new range of tasty and satisfying recipes, together with plenty of useful tips on how to shop and cook to best suit your fast days.

She has also put together a new section looking at motivation, based in part on what those who have tried the diet have told us.

The original book has sold in over forty-two countries, making intermittent fasting into a truly international phenomenon. Although there are many different forms of intermittent fasting (and we discuss most of them in this book), 5:2, a term that I used to describe my particular form (cutting your calories to one-quarter two days a week), is the one that people seem to find easiest to do and that has become the most firmly embedded in the national psyche.

We're told that 5:2 has been embraced by celebrities like Beyoncé and Benedict Cumberbatch; it has become the diet of choice for government ministers, for the Chancellor of the Exchequer, and for the former Governor of the Bank of England; and we have had grateful messages of thanks from doctors, surgeons, priests, business leaders, sports teachers, school heads, politicians, and a Nobel prizewinner.

We set up a website (thefastdiet.co.uk), which is thriving and whose members support others who are thinking of trying intermittent fasting with helpful advice and tips. I have learned a great deal from their experiences and questions.

The website contains thousands of success stories. These are a small sample:

"I heard the author on a radio show and he made so much sense I tried the diet. I have never stayed on a diet before. I lost 40 pounds in a few months. It is six months later and the weight is still gone."

"I've now lost about 19 pounds in 5 weeks, my body fat is down from 37 percent to 33 percent, and I can take my jeans off without undoing them, and I'm happy to do so if anyone will watch!"

"My body shape has changed beyond recognition. My muffin top has gone and I have gained a waist instead! I have been doing this for 21 weeks and have lost 19 pounds, as well as 3 inches off my waist, 3 inches off my hips, and 2 inches off each thigh. My psoriasis has gone too. I am 42 . . . and looking the best I have in 20 years."

Nothing works for everyone, and some people have struggled to make it work for them. We include an updated "troubleshooting" Q&A section to offer some helpful pointers to maximize your chances of success.

So Why Does It Work?

In the first half of this book, I delve into the science behind intermittent fasting. But one of the main reasons I think that the FastDiet has been so successful is psychological. When you are on the 5:2 diet, you aren't on a constant treadmill, dieting all the time.

I certainly find it easier to resist the temptation to eat a bar of chocolate by saying to myself, "I will have it tomorrow." Then tomorrow comes and maybe I eat it. But sometimes I don't.

Intermittent fasting also teaches you better ways of eating. If you follow our recipes and satisfy your hunger on fasting days by eating vegetables and good protein, then over time you'll discover that when you get hungry you are more likely to crave the healthy stuff. As someone recently wrote to me:

"You don't get cravings, you don't spend money on special foods or programs. I lost more than 25 pounds and my husband lost more than 35 pounds. It was easy to do, and we have maintained the weight loss, even over the holidays. I wish I had discovered this method 30 years ago."

The question I get asked most often is, not surprisingly,

"Are you still doing it?" The answer is, "yes and no." Back in the summer of 2012, I lost nearly 20 pounds, most of it fat, on the 5:2 diet. I also saw some spectacular improvements in things like my fasting glucose levels.

I didn't, however, want to go on losing weight, so I switched to doing mainly 6:1 (cutting my calories just one day a week). That, along with a regimen of FastExercise (which I describe in the second half of the book), has kept my weight stable for the last two years. Stable, that is, apart from Christmas and the occasional lapse.

I can honestly say I am in far better shape than I was two years ago, and I'm delighted so many other people have done likewise.

Like me, Mimi is following a 6:1 protocol, and the weight she lost in the first six months of the FastDiet (15 pounds) has stayed off for good. If there's a blowout for birthdays or holidays, she turns the dial back up to 5:2 and soon gets back on track. One of her greatest joys is her father's progress on the FastDiet: after decades of being overweight, he lost over 56 pounds in a single year—an astounding, life-changing achievement. As he says, "It's not like dieting at all; these days, I barely notice I'm doing it. Since New Year's Day, I can only remember being hungry once."

We both hope you enjoy this updated book and look forward to hearing more from you.

Michael Mosley, September 2015

Part One

THE

FastDiet

Introduction
to the FastDiet

OVER THE LAST FEW DECADES, FOOD FADS HAVE come and gone, but the standard medical advice on what constitutes a healthy lifestyle has stayed much the same: eat low-fat foods, exercise more . . . and never, ever skip meals. Over that same period, levels of obesity worldwide have soared.

Now many of those old certainties are being questioned.

When we first read about the benefits of intermittent fasting, we, like many, were skeptical. Fasting seemed drastic, difficult—and we both knew that dieting of any description is generally doomed to fail. But now that we've looked at it in depth and tried it ourselves, we are convinced of its remarkable potential. As one of the medical experts interviewed for this book puts it: "There is nothing else you can do to your body that is as powerful as fasting."

There is nothing else you can do to your body that is as powerful as fasting.

Fasting: An Ancient Idea, a Modern Method

Fasting is nothing new. As we'll discover in the next chapter, your body is designed to fast. We evolved at a time when food was scarce; we are the product of millennia of feast or famine. The reason we respond so well to intermittent fasting may be because it mimics, far more accurately than three meals a day, the environment in which modern humans were shaped.

Fasting, of course, remains an article of faith for many. The fasts of Lent, Yom Kippur, and Ramadan are just some of the better-known examples. Greek Orthodox Christians are encouraged to fast for 180 days of the year (according to Saint Nikolai of Zicha, "Gluttony makes a man gloomy and fearful, but fasting makes him joyful and courageous"), while Buddhist monks fast on the new moon and full moon of each lunar month.

Many more of us, however, seem to be eating most of the time. We're rarely ever hungry. But we *are* dissatisfied. With our weight, our bodies, our health.

Intermittent fasting can put us back in touch with our human selves. It is a route not only to weight loss, but also to long-term health and well-being. Scientists are only just beginning to discover and prove how powerful a tool it can be.

A review article recently published in the scientific journal *Cell Metabolism*, "Fasting: Molecular Mechanisms and Clinical Applications,"[1] which looks at some of the most recent human and animal studies, makes the point that "fasting has been practiced for millennia, but only recently, studies have shed light on its role in adaptive cellular responses that reduce oxidative damage and inflammation, optimize energy metabolism, and bolster cellular protection."

In other words, we now know, through proper scientific studies, that fasting reduces many of the things that promote aging ("oxidative damage and inflammation"), while increasing the body's ability to protect and repair itself ("cellular protection").

The article concludes that fasting "helps reduce obesity, hypertension, asthma, and rheumatoid arthritis. Thus, fasting has the potential to delay aging and help prevent and treat diseases."

This book is a product of cutting-edge scientific research and its impact on our current thinking about weight loss, disease resistance, and longevity. But it is also the result of our personal experiences.

Both are relevant here—the lab and the lifestyle—so we investigate intermittent fasting from two complementary perspectives. First, Michael, who used his body and medical training to test its potential, explains the scientific foundations of intermittent fasting (IF) and the 5:2 diet—something he brought to the world's attention during the summer of 2012.

Then Mimi offers a practical guide on how to do it safely, effectively, and in a sustainable way, a way that will fit easily into your normal everyday life. She looks in detail at how fasting feels, what you can expect from day to day, what to eat, and when to eat, and provides a host of tips and strategies to help you gain the greatest benefit from the diet's simple precepts.

As you'll see below, the FastDiet has changed both of our lives. We hope it will do the same for you.

Michael's Motivation: A Male Perspective

I am a 57-year-old male, and before I embarked on my exploration of intermittent fasting, I was mildly overweight: at five feet, eleven inches, I weighed around 187 pounds and had a body mass index of 26, which put me into the overweight category. Until my midthirties, I had been slim, but like many people I then gradually put on weight, around one pound a year. This doesn't sound like much, but over a couple of decades it pushed me up and up. Slowly I realized that I was starting to resemble my father, a man who struggled with weight all his life and died in his early seventies of complications associated with diabetes. At his funeral many of his friends commented on how like him I had become.

While making a documentary for the BBC, I was fortunate enough to have an MRI (magnetic resonance imaging) scan done. This revealed that I am a TOFI—thin on the outside, fat inside. This visceral fat is the most dangerous sort of fat, because it wraps itself around your internal organs and puts you at risk for heart disease and diabetes. I later had blood tests that showed I was heading toward diabetes, and had a cholesterol score that was also way too high. Obviously, I was going to have to do something about this. I tried following standard advice, except it made little difference. My weight and blood profile remained stuck in the "danger ahead" zone.

I had never tried dieting before because I'd never found a diet that I thought would work. I'd watched my father try every form of diet, from Scarsdale through Atkins, from the Cambridge Diet to the Drinking Man's Diet. He'd lost weight on each one of them, and then within a few months put it all back on, and more.

Then, at the beginning of 2012, I was approached by Aidan Laverty, editor of the BBC science series *Horizon*, who asked if I would like to put myself forward as a guinea pig to explore the science behind life extension. I wasn't sure what we would find, but along with producer Kate Dart and researcher Roshan Samarasinghe, we quickly focused on calorie restriction and fasting as a fruitful area to explore.

Calorie restriction (CR) is pretty brutal; it involves eating an awful lot less than a normal person would expect to eat, and doing so every day of your (hopefully) long life. The reason people put themselves through this is because it is the only intervention that has been shown to extend lifespan, at least in animals. There are around 50,000 CRONies (Calorie Restriction with Optimum Nutrition) worldwide, and I have met quite a number of them. Despite their generally fabulous biochemical profile, I have never been seriously tempted to join their skinny ranks. I simply don't have the willpower or desire to live permanently on an extreme low-calorie diet.

So I was delighted to discover intermittent fasting (IF),

which involves eating fewer calories, but *only some of the time*. If the science was right, it offered the benefits of CR but without the pain.

I set off around the United States, meeting leading scientists who generously shared their research and ideas with me. It became clear that IF was no fad. But it wouldn't be as easy as I'd originally hoped. As you'll see later in the book, there are many different forms of intermittent fasting. Some involve eating nothing for twenty-four hours or longer. Others involve eating a single, low-calorie meal once a day, every other day. I tried both but couldn't imagine doing either on a regular basis. I found it was simply too hard.

Instead I decided to create and test my own modified version. Five days a week, I would eat normally; on the remaining two I would eat a quarter of my usual calorie intake (that is, 600 calories).

I split the 600 calories in two—around 250 calories for breakfast and 350 calories for supper—effectively fasting for around twelve hours at a stretch. I also decided to split my fasting days: I would fast on Mondays and Thursdays. I became my own experiment.

The program, *Eat, Fast, Live Longer*, which detailed my adventures with what we were now calling the 5:2 diet, appeared on the BBC during the London Olympics in August 2012. I expected it to be lost in the media frenzy that surrounded the Games, but instead it generated a frenzy of its own. The program was watched by more than 2.5 million people—a huge audience for *Horizon*—and hundreds of thousands more on YouTube. My Twitter account,

@DrMichaelMosley, went into overdrive, my followers tripled; everyone wanted to try my version of intermittent fasting, and they were all asking me what they should do. The newspapers took up the story. Articles appeared in the *Times* (London), the *Daily Telegraph*, the *Daily Mail*, and the *Mail on Sunday*. Before long, it was picked up by newspapers all over the world—in New York, Los Angeles, Paris, Madrid, Montreal, Islamabad, and New Delhi. Online groups were created, menus and experiences swapped, chat rooms started buzzing about fasting. People began to stop me on the street and tell me how well they were doing on the 5:2 diet. They also e-mailed details of their experiences. Among those e-mails, a surprisingly large number were from doctors. Like me, they had initially been skeptical, but they had tried it for themselves, found that it worked, and had begun suggesting it to their patients. They wanted information, menus, details of the scientific research to scrutinize. They wanted me to write a book. I hedged, procrastinated, then finally found a collaborator, Mimi Spencer, whom I liked and trusted and who has an in-depth knowledge of food. Which is how what you are reading came about.

Mimi's Motivation: A Female Perspective

I started intermittent fasting on the day I was commissioned to write a feature for the *Times* about Michael's *Horizon* program. It was the first I'd heard of intermittent fasting, and the idea appealed immediately, even to a cynical soul who has spent two decades examining the curious acrobatics of the fashion industry, the beauty business, and the diet trade.

I'd dabbled in diets before—show me a forty-something woman who hasn't—losing weight, then losing faith within weeks and piling it all back on. Though never overweight, I'd long been interested in dropping that reluctant seven to ten pounds—the pounds I picked up in pregnancy and somehow never lost. The diets I tried were always too hard to follow, too complicated to implement, too boring, too tough, too single-strand, too invasive, sucking the juice out of life and leaving you with the scraps. There was nothing I found that I could adopt and thread into the context of my life—as a mother, a working woman, a wife.

I've argued for years that dieting is a fool's game, doomed to fail because of the restrictions and deprivations imposed on an otherwise happy life, but this felt immediately different. The scientific evidence was extensive and compelling, and (crucially for me) the medical community was positive. The effects, for Michael and others, were impressive, startling even. In his *Horizon* documentary, Michael called it the "beginning of something huge . . . which could radically transform the nation's health." I couldn't resist. Nor could I conceive of a reason to wait.

The scientific evidence was extensive and compelling, and (crucially for me) the medical community was positive.

In the two and a half years since I wrote the *Times* feature, I have remained a convert. An evangelist, actually. I'm still "on" the FastDiet now, following a 6:1 pattern, but I barely notice it. At the outset, I weighed 132 pounds. At five feet, seven inches, my BMI was an okay 21.4. Today, as I write, I weigh 119 pounds, with a BMI of 19.4. That's a weight off. I feel light, lean, and alive. Fasting has become part of my weekly life, something I do automatically without stressing about it.

These days, I have more energy, more bounce, clearer skin, a greater zest for life. And—it has to be said—new jeans (27-inch waist) and none of my annual bikini dread as summer approaches. But perhaps more important, I know that there's a long-term gain. I'm doing the best for my body and my brain. It's an intimate revelation, but one worth sharing.

> I feel light, lean, and alive.

The FastDiet: The Potential, the Promise

We know that for many people, the standard diet advice simply does not work. The FastDiet is a radical alternative. It has the potential to change the way we think about eating and weight loss.

★ The FastDiet demands that we think about not just *what* we eat, but *when* we eat it.

★ There are no complicated rules to follow; the strategy is flexible, comprehensible, and user-friendly.

★ There is no daily slog of calorie control—none of the boredom, frustration, or serial deprivation that characterizes conventional diet plans.

★ Yes, it involves fasting, but not as you know it; you won't "starve" on any given day.

★ You can still enjoy the foods you love—most of the time.

★ Once the weight is off, sticking to the basic program will mean that it stays off.

★ Weight loss is only one benefit of the FastDiet. The real dividend is the potential long-term health gains—cutting your risk of a range of diseases, including diabetes, heart disease, and cancer.

★ You will soon come to understand that it is not a diet. It is much more than that: it is a sustainable strategy for a healthy, long life.

Now you'll want to understand exactly how we can make these dramatic assertions. In the next chapter, Michael explains the science that makes the FastDiet tick.

CHAPTER ONE

The Science of Fasting

FOR MOST ANIMALS OUT IN THE WILD, PERIODS OF feast or famine are the norm. Our remote ancestors did not often eat four or five times a day. Instead they would kill, gorge, lie around, and then have to go for long periods of time without having anything to eat. Our bodies and our genes were forged in an environment of scarcity, punctuated by the occasional massive blowout.

These days, of course, things are very different. We eat all the time. Fasting—the voluntary abstaining from eating food—is seen as a rather eccentric, not to mention unhealthy, thing to do. Most of us expect to eat at least three meals a day and have substantial snacks in between. In between the meals and the snacks, we also graze: a milky cappuccino here, the odd cookie there, or maybe a smoothie because it's "healthier."

Once upon a time, parents told their children, "Don't

eat between meals." Those times are long gone. Recent research in the United States, which compared the eating habits of 28,000 children and 36,000 adults over the last thirty years, found that the amount of time between what the researchers coyly described as "eating occasions" has fallen by an average of an hour. In other words, over the last few decades the amount of time we spend "not eating" has dropped dramatically.[1] In the 1970s, adults would go about four and a half hours without eating, while children would be expected to last about four hours between meals. Now it's down to three and a half hours for adults and three hours for children, and that doesn't include all the drinks and nibbles.

The idea that eating little and often is a "good thing" has been driven partly by snack manufacturers and faddish diet books, but it has also had support from the medical establishment. Their argument is that it is better to eat lots of small meals because that way we are less likely to get hungry and gorge on high-fat junk. I can appreciate the argument, and there have been some studies that suggest there are health benefits to eating small meals regularly, as long as you don't simply end up eating more. Unfortunately, in the real world that's exactly what happens.

In the study I quoted above, the authors found that compared to thirty years ago, we not only eat around 180 calories a day more in snacks—much of it in the form of milky drinks, smoothies, carbonated beverages—but we also eat more when it comes to our regular meals, up by an average of 120 calories a day. In other words, snacking doesn't mean that we eat less at mealtimes; it just whets the appetite.

Do you need to eat lots of small meals to keep your metabolic rate high?

One of the other supposed benefits of eating lots of small meals is that it will increase your metabolic rate and help you lose weight. But is it true?

In a recent study, researchers at the Institute for Clinical and Experimental Medicine in Prague decided to test this idea by feeding two groups of type 2 diabetics meals with the same number of calories, but taken as either two or six meals a day.[2]

Both groups ate 1,700 calories a day. The "two meals a day group" ate their first meal between 6:00 a.m. and 10:00 a.m. and their next meal between noon and 4:00 p.m. The "snackers" ate their 1,700 calories as 6 meals, spread out at regular intervals throughout the day. Despite eating the same number of calories, the "two meal a day" group lost, on average, 3 pounds more than the snackers and about 1½ inches more around their waists.

Contrary to what you might expect, the volunteers eating their calories spread out as 6 meals a day felt less satisfied and hungrier than those sticking to the two meals. The lead scientist, Dr. Kahleova, believes cutting down to two meals a day could also help people without diabetes who are trying to lose weight.

So, simply cutting out snacks and one meal a day could be an effective weight-loss strategy. Yet eating throughout the day is now so normal, so much the expected thing to do, that it is almost shocking to suggest there is value in doing the absolute opposite. When I first started deliberately cutting back my calories two days a week, I discovered some unexpected things about myself, my beliefs, and my attitudes to food.

★ I discovered that I often eat when I don't need to. I do it because the food is there, because I am afraid that I will get hungry later, or simply from habit.

★ I assumed that when you get hungry, it builds and builds until it becomes intolerable, and so you bury your face in a vat of ice cream. I found instead that hunger passes, and once you have been really hungry, you no longer fear it.

★ I thought that fasting would make me distractible, unable to concentrate. What I've discovered is that it sharpens my senses and my brain.

I thought that fasting would make me
distractible, unable to concentrate.
What I've discovered is that it
sharpens my senses and my brain.

★ I wondered if I would feel faint for much of the time. It turns out the body is incredibly adaptable, and many athletes I've spoken to advocate training while fasting.

★ I feared it would be incredibly hard to do. It isn't.

Why I Got Started

Although most of the great religions advocate fasting (the Sikhs are an exception, although they do allow fasting for medical reasons), I have always assumed that this was principally a way of testing yourself and your faith. I could see potential spiritual benefits, but I was deeply skeptical about the physical benefits.

I have also had a number of body-conscious friends who, down the years, have tried to get me to fast, but I could never accept their explanation that the reason for doing so was "to rest the liver" or "to remove the toxins." Neither explanation made any sense to a medically trained skeptic like me. I remember one friend telling me that after a couple of weeks of fasting, his urine had turned black, proof that the toxins were leaving. I saw it as proof that he was an ignorant hippie and that whatever was going on inside his body as a result of fasting was extremely damaging.

As I wrote earlier, what convinced me to try fasting was a combination of my own personal circumstances—in my midfifties, with high blood sugar, slightly overweight—and the emerging scientific evidence, which I list below.

That Which Does Not Kill Us
Makes Us Stronger

There were a number of researchers who inspired me in different ways, but one who stands out is Dr. Mark Mattson of the National Institute on Aging in Bethesda, Maryland. A few years ago he wrote an article with Edward Calabrese in *New Scientist* magazine. Entitled "When a little poison is good for you,"[3] it really made me sit up and think.

"A little poison is good for you" is a colorful way of describing the theory of hormesis—the idea that when a human, or indeed any other creature, is exposed to a stress or toxin, it can toughen them up. Hormesis is not just a variant of "join the army and it will make a man of you"; it is now a well-accepted biological explanation of how things operate at the cellular level.

Take, for example, something as simple as exercise. When you run or pump iron, what you are actually doing is damaging your muscles, causing small tears and rips. If you don't completely overdo it, then your body responds by doing repairs, making the muscles stronger in the process.

Thinking or having to make decisions can also be stressful, yet there is good evidence that challenging yourself intellectually is good for your brain, and the reason it is good is because it produces changes in brain cells that are similar to the changes you see in muscle cells after exercise. The right sort of stress keeps us younger and smarter.

Vegetables are another example of the power of hormesis. We all know that we should eat lots of fruits and vegetables because they are chock full of antioxidants—and antioxidants are great because they mop up the dangerous free radicals that roam our bodies doing harm.

The trouble with this widely accepted explanation of how fruit and vegetables "work" is that it is almost certainly wrong, or at least incomplete. The levels of antioxidants in fruits and vegetables are far too low to have the profound effects they clearly do. In addition, the attempts to extract antioxidants from plants and then give them to us in a concentrated form as a health-inducing supplement have been unconvincing when tested in long-term trials. Beta carotene, when you get it in the form of a carrot, is undoubtedly good for you. When beta carotene was taken out of the carrot and given as a supplement to patients with cancer, it actually seemed to make them worse.

If we look through the prism of hormesis at the way vegetables work in our bodies, we can see that the reasons for their benefits are quite different.

Consider this apparent paradox: Bitterness is often associated in the wild with poison, something to be avoided. Plants produce a huge range of so-called phytochemicals, and some of them act as natural pesticides to keep mammals like us from eating them. The fact that they taste bitter is a clear warning signal: "keep away." So there are good evolutionary reasons why we should dislike and avoid bitter-tasting foods. Yet some of the vegetables that are particularly good for us, such as cabbage, cauliflower, broccoli, and other members of the genus *Brassica*, are so bitter that even as adults many of us struggle to love them.

The resolution to this paradox is that these vegetables taste bitter because they contain chemicals that are potentially poisonous. The reason they don't harm us is that these chemicals exist in vegetables at low doses that are not toxic. Instead they activate stress responses and switch on genes that protect and repair.

Once you start looking at the world in this way, you realize that many activities we initially find stressful—eating bitter vegetables, going for a run, intermittent fasting—are far from harmful. The challenge itself seems to be part of the benefit. The fact that prolonged starvation is clearly very bad for you does not imply that short periods of intermittent fasting must be a little bit bad for you. In fact the reverse is true.

This point was vividly made to me by Dr. Valter Longo, director of the University of Southern California's Longevity Institute. His research is mainly into the study of why we age, particularly concerning approaches that reduce the risk of developing age-related diseases such as cancer and diabetes.

I went to see Valter, not just because he is a world expert, but also because he had kindly agreed to act as my fasting mentor and buddy, to help inspire and guide me through my first experience of fasting.

Valter has not only been studying fasting for many years, he is also a keen adherent of it. He lives by his research and thrives on the sort of low-protein, high-vegetable diet that his grandparents enjoy in southern Italy. Perhaps not coincidentally, his grandparents live in a part of Italy that has an extraordinarily high concentration of long-lived people. As well as following a fairly strict diet, Valter skips lunch to keep his weight down. Beyond this, once every six months or so he does a prolonged fast that lasts several days. Tall, slim, energetic, and Italian, he is an inspiring poster boy for would-be fasters.

The main reason he is so enthusiastic about fasting is that his research, and that of others, has demonstrated the extraordinary range of measurable health benefits you get from doing it. Going without food for even quite short periods of time switches on a number of so-called repair genes, which, as he explained, can confer long-term benefits. "There is a lot of initial evidence to suggest that temporary periodic fasting can induce long-lasting changes that can be beneficial against aging and diseases," he told me. "You take a person, you fast them, after twenty-four hours everything is revolutionized. And even if you took a cocktail of drugs, very potent drugs, you will never even get close to what fasting does. The beauty of fasting is that it's all coordinated."

There is a lot of initial evidence to suggest
that temporary periodic fasting can
induce long-lasting changes that can be
beneficial against aging and diseases.

Fasting and Longevity

Most of the early long-term studies on the benefits of fasting were done on rodents. They gave us important insights into the molecular mechanisms that underpin fasting.

In one early study from 1945, mice were fasted for either one day in four, one day in three, or one day in two. The researchers found that the fasted mice lived longer than a control group, and that the more they fasted, the longer they lived. They also found that unlike calorie-restricted mice, the fasted mice were not physically stunted.[4]

Since then, numerous studies have confirmed, at least in rodents, the value of fasting. Not only does fasting extend their lifespan, but it also increases their "healthspan," the amount of time they live without chronic age-related diseases. Postmortems on rodents that have been calorie restricted show they have far fewer signs of cancer, heart disease, or neurodegeneration.

A recent article in the prestigious science journal *Nature* points to the wealth of research on the benefits of fasting, while at the same time noting sadly that so far "these insights have made hardly a dent in human medicine."[5] But why does fasting help? What is the mechanism?

Valter has access to his own supply of genetically engineered mice known as dwarf or Laron mice, which he was keen to show me. These mice, though small, hold the record for longevity extension in a mammal. In other words, they live for an astonishingly long time.

The average mouse doesn't live that long, perhaps two years. Laron mice live nearly twice that, many for almost four years when they are also calorie restricted. In a human, that would be the equivalent of reaching almost 170.

The fascinating thing about Laron mice is not just how long they live, but that they stay healthy for most of their very long lives. They simply don't seem to be prone to diabetes or cancer, and when they die, more often than not it is of natural causes. Valter told me that during an autopsy, it is often impossible to find a cause of death. The mice just seem to drop dead.

The reason these mice are so small and so long-lived is that they are genetically engineered so that their bodies do not respond to a hormone called IGF-1, insulin-like growth factor 1. IGF-1, as its name implies, has growth-promoting effects on almost every cell in the body. In other words, it keeps your cells constantly active. You need adequate levels of IGF-1 and other growth factors when you are young and growing, but high levels later in life appear to lead to accelerated aging and cancer. As Valter puts it, it's like driving along with your foot flat down on the accelerator pedal, pushing the car to continue to perform all the time. "Imagine, instead of occasionally taking your car to the garage and changing parts and pieces, you simply kept on driving it and driving it and driving it. Well, the car, of course, is going to break down."

Valter's work is focused on trying to figure out how you can go on driving as much as possible, and as fast as possible, while enjoying life. He thinks the answer is periodic fasting.

Because one of the ways fasting works is by making your body reduce the amount of IGF-1 it produces.

The evidence that IGF-1 plays a key role in many of the diseases of aging comes not just from engineered rodents like the Laron mice, but also from humans. For the last several years, Valter has been studying villagers in Ecuador with a genetic defect called Laron syndrome or Laron-type dwarfism. This is an extremely rare condition that affects fewer than 350 people in the entire world. People with Laron syndrome have a mutation in their growth hormone receptor (GHR) and very low levels of IGF-1. The genetically engineered Laron mice have a similar type of GHR mutation.

The villagers with Laron syndrome are normally quite short; many are less than four feet tall. The thing that is most surprising about them, however, is that like the Laron mice, they simply don't seem to develop common diseases like diabetes and cancer. In fact, Valter says that though they have been studied for many years, he has not come across a single case of someone with Laron dying of cancer. Yet their relatives, who live in the same household but who don't have Laron syndrome, do get cancer.

Disappointingly for anyone hoping that IGF-1 will provide the secrets of immortality, people with Laron syndrome—unlike the mice—are not that exceptionally long-lived. They certainly lead long lives, but not extremely long lives. Valter thinks one reason for this may be that they tend to enjoy life rather than worry about their lifestyle. "They smoke, eat a high-calorie diet, and then they look at me and they say, 'Oh, it doesn't matter, I'm immune.' "

Valter thinks they prefer the idea of living as they want and dying at age 85, rather than living more carefully and perhaps going beyond 100. He would like to persuade some of them to take on a healthier lifestyle and see what happens, but knows he wouldn't live long enough to see the outcome.

Fasting and Repair Genes

As well as reducing circulating levels of IGF-1, fasting also appears to switch on a number of repair genes. The reason this happens is not fully understood, but the evolutionary argument goes something like this: As long as we have plenty of food, our bodies are mainly interested in growing, having sex, and reproducing. Nature has no long-term plans for us; she does not invest in our old age. Once we've reproduced, we become disposable. So what happens if you decide to fast? Well, the body's initial reaction is one of shock. Signals go to the brain reminding you that you are hungry, urging you to go out and find something to eat. But you resist. The body now decides that the reason you are not eating as much and as frequently as you usually do must be because you are now in a famine situation. In the past this would have been quite normal.

In a famine situation, there is no point in expending energy on growth or sex. Instead, the wisest thing the body can do is to spend its precious store of energy on repair, trying to keep you in reasonable shape until the good times return once more. The result is that as well as removing its foot from the accelerator, your body takes itself along to the cellular equivalent of a garage. There, all the little gene mechanics are ordered to start doing some of the urgent maintenance tasks that have been put off till now.

One of the things that calorie restriction does, for example, is to switch on a process called autophagy.[6] Autophagy, meaning "self-eat," is a process by which the body breaks down and recycles old and tired cells. Just as with a car, it is important to get rid of damaged or aging parts if you are going to keep things in good working order.

Intermittent Fasting and Stem Cell Regeneration

Fasting not only helps clear out damaged old cells but can also spark the production of new ones. In a particularly fascinating study published in June 2014, Valter and his colleagues showed, for the first time, that fasting can switch on stem cells and regenerate the immune system.[7]

Stem cells are cells that, when activated, can grow into almost any other cell. They can become brain, liver, heart tissue, whatever. The reason that this recent study is so exciting is because one of the things that happens when you age is that your immune system tends to get weaker. Being able to create new white cells and a more powerful immune system will not only keep infections at bay but may also reduce your risk of developing cancer; mutating cells that could turn into a cancer are normally destroyed by the immune system long before they can escape and multiply.

There have been claims that fasting can harm your immune system and, initially, Valter's studies seemed to support this view, as he explains, "When you starve, your system tries to save energy, and one of the things it can do to save energy is to recycle a lot of the immune cells that are not needed, especially those that may be damaged. What we started noticing in both our human work and animal work is that the white blood cell count goes down with prolonged fasting."

Clearly in the long run this would be harmful, as a fall in white blood cells would make you more vulnerable to infections and to cancers. But, as we have seen with hormesis, just because something is bad for you when pushed to the extreme does not mean it is bad when done in moderation. Valter discovered, to his considerable surprise, that if you do a short fast and then eat, you get a rebound effect, with the creation of new, more active cells. "We could not have predicted," he said, "that fasting would have such a remarkable effect."

It seems that fasting not only clears out the old, damaged white blood cells and lowers levels of IGF-1, it also reduces the activity of a gene called PKA. PKA produces an enzyme that normally acts like a brake on regeneration. "PKA is the key gene that needs to be shut down in order for stem cells to switch into regenerative mode," Valter says.

Intermittent fasting seems to give the "okay" for stem cells to go ahead and begin proliferating. This research certainly suggests that if your immune system is not as effective as it was (either because you are older or because you have had a medical treatment such as chemotherapy), then periods of intermittent fasting may help regenerate it.

Michael Experiences a Four-Day Fast

Valter thinks that the majority of people with a BMI over 25 would benefit from fasting, but he also thinks that if you plan to do it for more than a day, it should be done in a proper center. As he puts it, "A prolonged fast is an extreme intervention. If it's done well, it can be very powerful in your favor. If it's done improperly, it can be very powerful against you." With a prolonged fast lasting several days, you also have a drop in blood pressure and some fairly profound metabolic reprogramming. Some people faint. It's not common, but it happens.

As Valter pointed out, the first time you try fasting for a few days, it can be a bit of a struggle. "Our bodies are used to high levels of glucose and high levels of insulin, so it takes time to adapt. But then eventually it's not that hard."

I wasn't keen to hear "eventually," but by then I knew I would have to give it a go. It was a challenge, and one I thought I could win. Brain against stomach. No contest. I had recently had my IGF-1 levels measured, and they were high. Not super high, as he kindly put it, but at the top end of the range (see my data on page 64).

High levels of IGF-1 are associated with a range of cancers, among them prostate cancer, which troubled my father. Would a four-day fast change anything?

I had been warned that the first few days might be tough, but after that I would start feeling the effects of a rush of what Valter termed well-being chemicals. Even better, the next time I fasted would be easier, because my body and brain would have a memory of it and understand what it was I was going through.

Having decided that I would try an extended fast, my next decision was how harsh to make it. A number of different countries have a tradition of fasting. The Russians seem to prefer it tough. For them, a fast consists of nothing but water, cold showers, and exercise. The Germans, on the other hand, prefer their fasts to be considerably gentler. Go to a fasting clinic in Germany and you will probably be fed around 200 calories a day in comfortable surroundings.

I wanted to see results, so I went for a British compromise. I would eat 25 calories a day, no cold showers, and just try working normally.

So on a warm Monday evening I enjoyed my last meal, an extremely filling dinner of steak, fries, and salad, washed down with beer. I felt a certain trepidation as I realized that for the next four days I would be drinking nothing but water, sugarless black tea, and coffee, and eating one measly cup of low-calorie soup a day.

Despite what I'd been told and read, before I began my fast I secretly feared that hunger would grow and grow, gnawing away inside me until I finally gave in and ran amok in a cake shop. The first twenty-four hours were quite tough, just as Valter had predicted, but as he also predicted, things got better, not worse. Yes, there were hunger pangs, sometimes quite distracting, but if I kept busy they went away.

During the first twenty-four hours of a fast there are some very profound changes going on inside the body. Within a few hours, glucose circulating in the blood is consumed. If that's not being replaced by food, then the body turns to glycogen, a stable form of glucose that is stored in the muscles and liver.

> During the first twenty-four hours of a fast there are some very profound changes going on inside the body.

Only when that's gone does it really switch on fat burning. What actually happens is that fatty acids are broken down in the liver, resulting in the production of something called ketone bodies. These ketone bodies are now used by the brain instead of glucose as a source of energy.

The first two days of a fast can be uncomfortable because your body and brain are having to cope with the switch from using glucose and glycogen as a fuel to using ketone bodies. The body is not used to them, so you can get headaches, though I didn't. You may find it hard to sleep. I didn't. The biggest problem I had with fasting is hard to put into words; it was sometimes just feeling "uncomfortable." I can't really describe it more accurately than that. I didn't feel faint, I just felt out of place.

I did, occasionally, feel hungry, but most of the time I was surprisingly cheerful. By day three the feel-good hormones had come to my rescue.

By Friday, day four, I was almost disappointed that it was ending. Almost. Despite Valter's warning that it would be unwise to gorge immediately upon breaking a fast, I got myself a plate of bacon and eggs and settled down to eat. After a few mouthfuls I was full. I really didn't need any more and in fact skipped lunch.

That afternoon I had myself tested again and discovered I had lost just under three pounds of body weight, a significant portion of which was fat. I was also happy to see that my blood glucose levels had fallen substantially and that my IGF-1 levels, which had been right at the top end of the recommended range, had gone right down. In fact, they had almost halved. This was all good news. I had lost some fat, my blood results were looking good, and I had learned that I can control my hunger. Valter was extremely pleased with these changes, particularly the fall in IGF-1, which he said would significantly reduce my risk of cancer. But he also warned me that if I went back to my old lifestyle, these changes would not be permanent.

Valter's research points toward the fact that high levels of protein, the amounts found in a typical Western diet, help keep IGF-1 levels high. I knew that there is protein in foods like meat and fish, but I was surprised there is so much in milk. I used to like drinking a skinny latte most mornings. I had the illusion that because it is made of skim milk, it is healthy. Unfortunately, though low in fat, a large latte comes in at around 11 grams of protein. The recommendation is that you stick to government guidelines, which can be found at websites like http://www.cdc.gov/nutrition

/everyone/basics/protein.html. Recommended levels vary according to age and gender. They are around 46 grams of protein for women between 19 and 75, and 55 grams of protein for men between 19 and 75. I realized that the lattes would have to go.

Fasting and Weight Loss

I did the four-day fast, as described above, mainly because I was curious. I would not recommend it as a weight-loss regimen because it is completely unsustainable. Unless they combine it with vigorous exercise, people who go on prolonged fasts lose muscle as well as fat. Then, when they stop (as they must eventually do), the risk is they will pile the weight right back on.

Fortunately, less drastic, intermittent fasting, the subject of this book, leads to steady weight loss, which seems to be both sustainable and without muscle loss.

ADF, Alternate-Day Fasting

One of the most extensively studied forms of short-term fasting is alternate-day fasting. As its name implies, it means you eat no food, or relatively little food, every other day. Dr. Krista Varady of the University of Illinois at Chicago has done a lot of the more recent studies in this area.

Krista is slim, charming, and very amusing. We first met

in an old-fashioned American diner, where I guiltily ate a burger and fries while Krista told me about the work she has been doing with human volunteers.[8] The version of ADF she has been testing is one where on fast days volunteers are allowed 25 percent of their normal energy needs, so men are allowed around 600 calories a day; women, 500 calories a day. On her regimen they eat all their calories in one go, at lunch. On their feed days they are asked to consume 125 percent of their normal energy needs.

Krista has done a number of studies on ADF, and what surprised her is that, although they are allowed to, people don't go crazy on their nonfast days. "I thought when I started running these trials that people would eat 175 percent the next day; they'd just fully compensate and wouldn't lose any weight. But most people eat around 110 percent, just slightly over what they usually eat. I haven't measured it yet, but I think it involves stomach size, how far that can expand out. Because eating almost twice the amount of food that you normally eat is actually pretty difficult. You can do it over time; people who are obese, their stomachs get bigger to accommodate, you know, 5,000 calories a day. But just to do it right off is actually pretty difficult."

In her earlier studies, the subjects were asked to stick to a low-fat diet, but what Krista wanted to know was whether ADF would also work if her subjects were allowed to eat a typical American high-fat diet. So she asked thirty-three obese volunteers, most of them women, to go on ADF for eight weeks. Before starting, the volunteers were divided into two groups. One group was put on a low-fat diet, eating low-fat cheeses and dairy, very lean meats, and a lot of fruit and vegetables. The other group was allowed to eat high-fat lasagna, pizza, the sort of diet a typical American might consume. Americans consume somewhere between 35 and 45 percent fat in their diet.

As Krista explained, the results were unexpected. The researchers and the volunteers had assumed that the people on the low-fat diet would lose more weight than those on the high-fat diet. But if anything, it was the other way around. The volunteers on the high-fat diet lost an average of 12.32 pounds, while those on the low-fat diet lost 9.24 pounds. They both lost about 2¾ inches around their waists.

Krista thinks that the main reason this happened was compliance. The volunteers randomized to the high-fat diet were more likely to stick to it than those on the low-fat diet simply because they found it a lot more palatable. And it wasn't just weight loss. Both groups saw impressive drops in LDL cholesterol (the bad cholesterol) and in blood pressure. This meant that they had reduced their risk of cardiovascular disease, of having a heart attack or stroke.

Krista doesn't want to encourage people to binge on junk food. She would much rather that people on ADF increase their intake of fruit and vegetables. The trouble is, as she pointed out rather exasperatedly, doctors have been encouraging people to embrace a healthy lifestyle for decades, and not enough of us are doing it. She thinks dietitians should take into account what people actually do rather than what we would like them to do.

One other significant benefit of intermittent fasting is

that you don't seem to lose muscle, which you would on a normal calorie-restricted regimen. Krista herself is not sure why that is and wants to do further research.

The Two-Day Fast

If you want to lose weight fast, then ADF is an effective, scientifically proven way to do it. The problem with ADF, which is why I personally am not so keen on it, is that you have to do it every other day.

In my experience this can be socially inconvenient as well as emotionally demanding. There is no pattern to your week and other people, friends, and family, find it hard to keep track of when your fast and feed days are.

Unlike Krista's subjects, I was not particularly overweight to start with, so I also worried about losing too much weight too rapidly. That is why, having tried ADF for a short while, I decided to cut back to fasting two days a week.

I now have my own experience of this to fall back on (see page 59), together with the experiences of thousands of others who have written to me over the last two years. But what trials have been done on two-day fasts in humans?

Dr. Michelle Harvie, a dietitian based at the Genesis Breast Cancer Prevention Centre at the Wythenshawe Hospital in Manchester, England, has done a number of studies assessing the effects of a two-day fast on female volunteers. In one study, she divided 115 women into three groups. One group was asked to stick to a 1,500-calorie Mediterranean diet, and was also encouraged to avoid high-fat foods and alcohol.[9] Another group was asked to eat normally five days a week, but to eat a 650-calorie, low-carbohydrate diet on the other two days. A final group was asked to avoid carbohydrates for two days a week, but was otherwise not calorie restricted.

After three months, the women on the two-day diet had lost an average of 8.1 pounds of fat, which was almost twice as much as the full-time dieters, who had lost an average of just 4.4 pounds of fat. Insulin resistance had also improved significantly in the two-day diet groups (see more on insulin on page 47). Those who stuck with the two-day diet for six months lost an average of 17 pounds and 3 inches from their waists. Some lost over 45 pounds.

The focus of Michelle's work is trying to reduce breast cancer risk through dietary interventions. Being obese and having high levels of insulin resistance are both risk factors. On the Genesis website (www.genesisuk.org), she points out that they have been studying intermittent fasting at the Genesis Breast Cancer Prevention Centre, University Hospital of South Manchester NHS Foundation Trust, for over eight years and that their research has shown that cutting down on your calories for two days a week gives the same benefits, possibly more, than by going on a normal calorie-restricted diet. "To date, our research has concluded that intermittent diets appear to be a safe, viable, alternative approach to weight loss and maintaining a lower weight, in comparison to daily dieting."

Another, more recent study looked at the effects on mood of being on a two-day diet.[10]

In this study, from Malaysia, thirty-two healthy males with an average age of 60 were randomly allocated to either a Sunnah (Muslim) fast, which meant cutting their calories on a Monday and a Thursday, or to a control group. They were then followed for three months.

Their mood was assessed using something called "The Profile of Mood States" questionnaire. The researchers found that not only did the intermittent fasting group lose far more fat than the control group, but that they felt much better on it. The researchers found that those doing intermittent fasting reported "significant decreases in tension, anger, confusion, and total mood disturbance, and improvements in vigor."

On an anecdotal level, I have heard very good things from those who have tried intermittent fasting. Many people find it surprisingly easy, others struggle, but generally things improve after the first couple of weeks. As one faster says, "I used to have mood swings as well as headaches; it does pass as you get used to this new way of eating. I found by week six it had become part of my routine."

To date, our research has concluded that intermittent diets appear to be a safe, viable, alternative approach to weight loss and maintaining a lower weight, in comparison to daily dieting.

Is It Just Calories?

If you eat 500 or 600 calories two days a week and don't significantly overcompensate during the rest of the week, then you will lose weight in a steady fashion.

I recently came across one particularly fascinating study suggesting that when you eat can be almost as important as what you eat.

In this study, scientists from the Salk Institute for Biological Studies took two groups of mice and fed them a high-fat diet.[11] All the mice got exactly the same amount of food to eat, the only difference being that the mice in one group were allowed to eat whenever they wanted, nibbling away when they were in the mood, rather like we do, while the mice in the other group had to eat their food within an eight-hour time period. This meant that there were sixteen hours of the day in which they were, involuntarily, fasting.

After 100 days, there were some truly dramatic differences between the two groups of mice. The mice who nibbled away at their fatty food had developed high cholesterol and high blood glucose, and had liver damage. The mice that had been forced to fast for sixteen hours a day put on far less weight (28 percent less) and suffered much less liver damage, despite having eaten exactly the same amount and quality of food. They also had lower levels of chronic inflammation, which suggests they had reduced risk of a number of diseases including heart disease, cancer, stroke, and Alzheimer's.

The Salk researchers' explanation for this is that all the

time you are eating, your insulin levels are elevated and your body is stuck in fat-storing mode (see the discussion of insulin on page 47). Only after a few hours of fasting is your body able to turn off the fat-storing and turn on the fat-burning mechanisms. So if you are a mouse and you are continually nibbling, your body will just continue making and storing fat, resulting in obesity and liver damage.

I think there is strong evidence that fasting offers multiple health benefits, as well as helping to achieve weight loss. I had been aware of some of these claims before I got really interested in fasting and, though initially skeptical, I was converted by the sheer weight of evidence.

But there was one area of study that was a complete surprise: research showing how fasting can improve mood and protect the brain from dementia and cognitive decline. This, for me, was something new, unexpected, and hugely exciting.

> But there was one area of study that was a complete surprise: research showing how fasting can improve mood and protect the brain from dementia and cognitive decline.

Fasting and the Brain

The brain, as Woody Allen once said, is my second favorite organ. I might even put it first, as without it nothing else would function. The brain, around three pounds of pinkish-grayish gunk with the consistency of tapioca, has been described as the most complex object in the known universe. It allows us to build, write poetry, dominate the planet, and even understand ourselves, something no other creature has succeeded in doing.

It is also an extremely efficient energy-saving machine, doing all that complicated thinking and making sure our bodies are functioning properly while using the same amount of energy as a 25-watt lightbulb. The fact that our brains are normally so flexible and adaptable makes it even more tragic when they go wrong. I am aware that as I get older my memory has become more fallible. I've compensated by using a range of memory tricks I've picked up over the years, but even so, I find myself occasionally struggling to remember names and dates. Far worse than this, however, is the fear that one day I may lose my mind entirely, perhaps developing some form of dementia. Obviously I want to preserve my brain in as good a shape as possible and for as long as possible. Fortunately fasting seems to offer significant protection.

The man I went to discuss my brain with was Mark Mattson.

Mark, a professor of neuroscience at the National Institute on Aging, is one of the most revered scientists in his field, the study of the aging brain. I find his work genuinely inspiring—suggesting, as it does, that fasting can help combat diseases like Alzheimer's, dementia, and memory loss.

Although I could have taken a taxi to his office, I chose to walk. I'm a fan of walking. It not only burns calories, it also improves the mood, and it may also help you retain your memory. Normally, as we get older, our brain shrinks, but one study found that in regular walkers the hippocampus, the area of the brain essential for memory, actually expanded.[12] Regular walkers have brains that in MRI scans look, on average, two years younger than the brains of those who are sedentary.

Mark, who studies Alzheimer's, lost his own father to dementia. He told me that although it didn't directly motivate him to go into this particular line of research—when he started his work on Alzheimer's disease, his father had not yet been diagnosed—it did give him insight into the condition.

Alzheimer's affects around 26 million people worldwide, and the problem will grow as the population ages. New approaches are desperately needed because the tragedy of Alzheimer's disease and other forms of dementia is that once you're diagnosed, it may be possible to delay, but not prevent, the inevitable deterioration. You are likely to get progressively worse to the point where you need constant care for many years. By the end, you may not even recognize the faces of those you once loved.

Can Fasting Make You Smarter?

Just as Valter Longo had, Mark took me off to see some mice. Like Valter's mice, these were genetically engineered, but Mark's mice had been modified to make them more vulnerable to Alzheimer's. The mice I saw were in a maze that they had to navigate in order to find food. Some of the mice performed this task with relative ease; others got disorientated and confused. This task and others like it are designed to reveal signs that the mice are developing memory problems; a mouse that is struggling will quickly forget which arm of the maze it has already traveled down.

If put on a normal diet, the genetically engineered Alzheimer's mice will quickly develop dementia. By the time they are a year old, the equivalent of middle age in humans, they normally have obvious learning and memory problems. The animals put on an intermittent fast, something Mark prefers to call "intermittent energy restriction," often go for up to twenty months without any detectable signs of dementia.[13] They only really start deteriorating toward the end of their lives. That's the equivalent in a human of the difference between developing signs of Alzheimer's at the age of 50 and the age of 80. I know which I would prefer.

Disturbingly, when these mice are put on a typical junk-food diet, they go downhill much earlier than even normally fed mice. "We put mice on a high-fat and high-fructose diet," Mark said, "and that has a dramatic effect; the animals have an earlier onset of the learning and memory problems, more accumulation of amyloid, and more problems with finding their way in a maze test."

In other words, junk food makes these mice fat and stupid.

One of the key changes that occurs in the brains of Mark's fasting mice is increased production of a protein called brain-derived neurotrophic factor. BDNF has been shown to stimulate stem cells to turn into new nerve cells in the hippocampus. As I mentioned earlier, this is a part of the brain that is essential for normal learning and memory.

But why should the hippocampus grow in response to fasting? Mark points out that from an evolutionary perspective it makes sense. After all, the times when you need to be smart and on the ball are when there's not a lot of food lying around. "If an animal is in an area where there's limited food resources, it's important that they are able to remember where food is, remember where hazards are, predators and so on. We think that people in the past who were able to respond to hunger with increased cognitive ability had a survival advantage."

We don't know for sure if humans grow new brain cells in response to fasting; to be absolutely certain, researchers would need to put volunteers on an intermittent fast and then kill them, take their brains out, and look for signs of new neural growth. It seems unlikely that many would volunteer for such a project. But researchers are doing a study in which volunteers fast and then MRI scans are used to see if the size of their hippocampi has changed over time.

As I mentioned above, these techniques have been used in humans to show that regular exercise, such as walking, increases the size of the hippocampus. Hopefully, similar studies will show that two days a week of intermittent fasting are good for learning and memory. On a purely anecdotal level, and using a sample size of one, it seems to work. Before starting the FastDiet, I did a sophisticated memory test online. Two months in I repeated the test, and my performance had, indeed, improved. If you are interested in doing something similar, then I suggest you go to cognitivefun.net/test/2. Let us know how it works out.

Fasting and Mood

One of the things that Valter Longo and others told me before I began my four-day fast was that it would be tough initially, but that after a while I would start to feel more cheerful, which was indeed what happened. Similarly, I was surprised to discover how positive I have felt while doing intermittent fasting. I expected to feel tired and crabby on my fasting days, but that didn't happen at all. So is this improved mood simply a psychological effect—that people who do intermittent fasting and lose weight feel good about themselves—or are there also chemical changes that are influencing mood?

According to Mark Mattson, one of the reasons people may find intermittent fasting relatively easy to do is because of its effects on brain-derived neurotrophic factor. BDNF not only seems to protect the brain against the ravages of dementia and age-related mental decline, but it may also improve your mood.

There have been a number of studies going back many years that suggest rising levels of BDNF have an antidepressant effect; at least they do in rodents. In one study, researchers injected BDNF directly into the brains of rats and found this had similar effects to repeated use of a standard antidepressant.[14] Another paper found that electroshock therapy, which is known to be effective in severe depression in human patients, seems to work, at least in part, because it stimulates the production of higher levels of BDNF.[15]

Mark Mattson believes that within a few weeks of starting a two-day-a-week fasting regimen, BDNF levels will start to rise, suppressing anxiety and elevating mood. He doesn't currently have the human data to fully support this claim, but he is doing trials on volunteers in which, among other things, his team is collecting regular samples of cerebrospinal fluid (the liquid that bathes the brain and spinal cord) in order to measure the changes that occur during intermittent fasts. This is not a trial for the fainthearted, as it requires regular spinal taps, but as Mark pointed out to me, many of his volunteers are already undergoing early signs of cognitive change, so they are extremely motivated.

Mark is keen to study and promote the benefits of intermittent fasting, as he is genuinely worried about the likely effects of the current obesity epidemic on our brains and our society. He also thinks that if you are considering intermittent fasting, you should get going sooner rather than later: "The age-related cognitive decline in Alzheimer's disease, the events that are occurring in the brain at the level of the nerve cells and the molecules in the nerve cells, those changes are occurring very early, probably decades before the subject starts to have learning and memory problems. That's why it's critical to start dietary regimens early on, when people are young or middle-aged, so that they can slow down the development of these processes in the brain and live to be ninety with their brain functioning perfectly well."

Like Mark, I'm convinced the human brain benefits from short periods abstaining from food. This is an exciting and fast-emerging area of research that many will watch with great interest. Beyond the brain, though, intermittent fasting also has measurable, beneficial effects on other areas in the body—on the heart, on blood profile, on cancer risk. And that's where we'll turn now.

> Beyond the brain, though, intermittent fasting also has measurable, beneficial effects on other areas in the body—on the heart, on blood profile, on cancer risk.

Fasting and the Heart

One of the main reasons I decided to try fasting was that I had tests suggesting I was heading for serious problems with my cardiovascular system. Nothing had happened yet, but the warning signs were flashing amber. The tests showed that my blood levels of LDL (low-density lipoprotein, the "bad" cholesterol) were disturbingly high, as were the levels of my fasting glucose.

To measure fasting glucose, you have to fast overnight, then give a sample of blood. The normal, desirable range is 3.9 to 5.8 mmol/l. Mine was 7.3 mmol/l. Diabetic, but not yet dangerously high. There are many reasons that you should do all you can to avoid becoming a diabetic, not the least the fact that it dramatically increases your risk of having a heart attack or stroke.

Fasting glucose is an important thing to measure because it is an indicator that all may not be well with your insulin levels.

Insulin: The Fat-Making Hormone

Insulin is a hormone that has a similar molecular structure to IGF-1, and like IGF-1 it tends to increase cell turnover and reduce autophagy (clearing up of old cells). But insulin is best known as a hormone that regulates blood sugar.

When we eat food, particularly foods rich in carbohydrates, our blood glucose levels rise and the pancreas, an organ tucked away below the ribs next to the left kidney, starts to churn out insulin. Glucose is the main fuel that our cells use for energy, but high levels of glucose circulating in the blood are toxic to your cells. The job of insulin, a hormone, is to regulate blood glucose levels, ensuring that they are neither too high nor too low. It normally does this with great precision. The problem comes when the pancreas gets overloaded.

Insulin is a sugar controller; it aids the extraction of glucose from blood and then stores it in places like your liver or muscles in a stable form called glycogen, to be used when and if it is needed. What is less commonly known is that insulin is also a fat controller. It inhibits something called lipolysis, the breakdown of stored body fat. At the same time, it forces fat cells to take up and store fat from your blood.

Insulin makes you fat. High levels lead to increased fat storage, low levels to fat depletion.

The trouble with constantly eating lots of sugary, carbohydrate-rich foods and drinks, as we increasingly do, is that this requires the release of more and more insulin to deal with the glucose surge. Up to a point, your pancreas will cope by simply pumping out ever-larger quantities of insulin. This leads to greater fat deposition and also increases cancer risk. Naturally enough, this can't go on forever. If you continue to produce ever-larger quantities of insulin, your cells will eventually rebel and become resistant to its effects. It's rather like shouting at your children; you can keep escalating things, but after a certain point they will simply stop listening.

Eventually the cells stop responding to insulin; your blood glucose levels now stay permanently high, and you will find you have joined the 285 million people around the world who have type 2 diabetes, a massive and rapidly growing problem worldwide. Over the last twenty years, numbers have risen almost tenfold, and there is no obvious sign that this trend is slowing.

Diabetes is associated with an increased risk of heart attack, stroke, impotence, blindness, and amputation due to poor circulation. It is also associated with brain shrinkage and dementia. Not a pretty picture.

One way to prevent the downward spiral into diabetes is to do more exercise and eat foods that do not lead to such big spikes in blood glucose and that do not have such a dramatic effect on insulin levels. More on this later. The other way is to try intermittent fasting.

How Intermittent Fasting Affects Insulin Sensitivity and Diabetes

In a study published in 2005, eight healthy young men were asked to fast every other day, twenty hours a day, for two weeks.[16] On their fasting days they were allowed to eat until 10:00 p.m., then not eat again until 6:00 p.m. the following evening. They were also asked to eat heartily the rest of the time to make sure they did not lose any weight.

The idea behind the experiment was to test the so-called thrifty hypothesis, the idea that since we evolved at a time of feast or famine, the best way to eat is to mimic those times. At the end of the two weeks, there were no changes in the volunteers' weight or body fat composition, which is what the researchers had intended. There was, however, a big change in their insulin sensitivity. In other words, after just two weeks of intermittent fasting, the same amount of circulating insulin now had a much greater effect on the volunteers' ability to store glucose or break down fat.

The researchers wrote jubilantly that "by subjecting healthy men to cycles of feast and famine we changed their metabolic status for the better." They also added that "to our knowledge this is the first study in humans in which an increased insulin action on whole body glucose uptake and adipose tissue lipolysis has been obtained by means of intermittent fasting."

One of the ways that intermittent fasting seems to improve insulin sensitivity is by forcing the body to break down fat cells and use the fat as an energy source. Researchers at the Intermountain Heart Institute in Utah reported at a recent meeting of the American Diabetes Association that after ten to twelve hours without food, the body starts looking for new energy sources. At the same time, it starts drawing LDL cholesterol from cells, possibly using it as fuel.

> By subjecting healthy men to cycles of feast and famine we changed their metabolic status for the better.

Dr. Benjamin Horne, director of the Institute, says that because fat cells are a major contributor to insulin resistance (when the body stops responding to insulin), breaking down fat cells may reduce the risk of diabetes developing. Short-term fasting also makes the cells of the body go into self-protection mode, where they become resensitized to insulin.

"Although fasting may protect against diabetes," Dr. Horne cautions, "it's important to keep in mind that these results are not instantaneous. It takes time. How long and how often people should fast for health benefits are additional questions we're just beginning to examine."

I don't know what impact intermittent fasting has had on my insulin sensitivity—it's a test that is hard to do and extremely expensive—but what I do know is that the effects on my blood sugar have been spectacular. Before I started intermittent fasting, my blood glucose level was 7.3 mmol/l, well above the acceptable range of 3.9 to 5.8 mmol/l. The last time I had my level measured it was 5.0 mmol/l, still a bit high but well within the normal range.

This is an incredibly impressive response. My doctor, who was preparing to put me on medication, was astonished at such a dramatic turnaround. Doctors routinely recommend a healthy diet to patients with high blood glucose, but it usually makes only a marginal difference. Intermittent fasting could have a game-changing effect on the nation's health.

Fasting and Cancer

My father was a lovely man but not a particularly healthy one. Overweight for much of his life, by the time he reached his sixties he had developed not only diabetes but also prostate cancer. He had an operation to remove the prostate cancer, which left him with embarrassing urinary problems. Understandably, I am not at all keen to go down that road.

My four-day fast, under Valter Longo's supervision, had shown me that it was possible to dramatically cut my IGF-1 (insulin-like growth factor 1) levels and by doing so, hopefully, my prostate cancer risk. I later discovered that by doing intermittent fasting and being a bit more careful with my protein intake, I could keep my IGF-1 down at healthy levels. The link between growth, fasting, and cancer is worth unpacking.

The cells in our bodies are constantly multiplying, replacing dead, worn out, or damaged tissue. This is fine as long as cellular growth is under control, but sometimes a cell mutates, grows uncontrollably, and turns into a cancer. Very high levels of a cellular stimulant like IGF-1 in the blood are likely to increase the chance of this happening.

When a cancer goes rogue, the normal options are surgery, chemotherapy, or radiation. Surgery is used to try to remove the tumor; chemotherapy and radiation are used to try to poison it. The major problem with chemotherapy and radiation is that they are not selective; as well as killing tumor cells they will also kill or damage surrounding healthy cells. They are particularly likely to damage rapidly dividing cells such as hair roots, which is why hair commonly falls out following therapy.

As I mentioned above, Valter Longo has shown that when we are deprived of food for even quite short periods of time, our body responds by slowing things down, going into repair and survival mode until food is once more abundant. That is true of normal cells. But cancer cells follow their own rules. They are, almost by definition, not under control and will go on selfishly proliferating whatever the circumstances. This "selfishness" creates an opportunity. At least in theory, if you fast just before chemotherapy, you create a situation in which your normal cells are hibernating while the cancer cells are running amok and are therefore more vulnerable.

In a paper published in 2008, Valter and colleagues showed that fasting "protects normal but not cancer cells against high-dose chemotherapy,"[17] followed by another paper in which they showed that fasting increased the efficacy of chemotherapy drugs against a variety of cancers.[18] Again, as is so often the case, this was a study done in mice.

But the implications of Valter's work were not missed by an eagle-eyed administrative judge named Nora Quinn, who saw a short article about it in the *Los Angeles Times*.

Nora's Story

I met Nora in Los Angeles. She is a feisty woman with a terrific, dry sense of humor. Nora first noticed she had a problem when, one morning, she put her hand on her breast and felt a lump the size of a walnut under her skin. After indulging, as she put it, in the fantasy that it was a cyst, she went to the doctor; it was removed and sent to a pathologist.

"The reality of your life always comes out in pathology," she told me. When the pathology report came back, it said that she had invasive breast cancer. She had a course of radiation and was about to start chemotherapy when she read about Valter's work with mice.

She tried to speak to Valter, but he wouldn't advise her because, up to that point, none of the trials he had run had been done with humans. He didn't know if it was safe for someone about to undergo chemo to fast, and he certainly wasn't going to encourage people like Nora to give it a go.

Undeterred, Nora did her own research and decided to try fasting for seven and a half days, before, during, and after her first bout of chemotherapy. Having discovered how tough it can be to do even a four-day fast while fully healthy, I'm surprised she was able to go through with it, though Nora says it's not so hard and I'm just a wimp. The results were mixed.

"After the first chemo I didn't get that sick, but my hair fell out, so I thought it wasn't working." So next time she didn't fast, and she was only medium sick. "I thought, seven and a half days of fasting to avoid being medium sick, this is a really bad deal. I am so not doing that again." So when it was time for her third course of chemo, she didn't fast. That, she now feels, was a mistake. "I got sick. I don't have words for how sick I was. I was weak, felt poisoned, and I couldn't get up. I felt like I was moving through Jell-O. It was absolutely horrible."

The cells that line the gut, like hair root cells, grow rapidly because they need to be constantly replaced. Chemotherapy can kill those cells, which is one reason that it can make people feel really ill.

By the time Nora had to undergo her fourth course of chemo, she had decided to try fasting once again. This time things went much better and she made a good recovery. She is currently cancer free.

Nora is convinced she benefited from fasting, but it's hard to be sure because she wasn't part of a proper medical trial. Valter and his colleagues at USC did, however, study what happened to her and ten other patients with cancer who had also decided to put themselves on a fast.[19] All of them reported fewer and less severe symptoms after chemotherapy, and most of them, including Nora, saw improvements in their blood results. The white cells and platelets, for example, recovered more rapidly when they had chemo while they were fasting than when they did not.

But why did Nora go rogue? Why didn't she fast under proper supervision? She says: "I decided to fast based on years of information from animal testing. I do agree that if you are going to do crazy things like I did, you should have medical supervision. But how? None of my doctors would listen to me."

Nora's self-experiment could have gone wrong, which is just one reason why such maverick behavior is not recommended. Her experience, however, and that of the other nine cancer patients, helped inspire further studies. For example, Valter and his colleagues have recently completed phase one of a clinical trial to see if fasting around the time of chemotherapy is safe—which it seems to be. The next phase is to assess whether it makes a measurable difference. At least ten other hospitals around the world are either doing or have agreed to do clinical trials. Go to our website, www.thefastdiet.co.uk, for the latest updates.

Fasting and Chronic Inflammation

IF and Asthma

One of the other unexpected benefits of intermittent fasting is its effects on allergic diseases such as asthma and eczema. These are autoimmune diseases, the result of an overactive immune system that is mistakenly attacking the body's own cells. You might imagine that if intermittent fasting leads to new, more active white blood cells then this in turn could make your asthma worse. Far from it. On our website several people have reported seeing improvements in their asthma since going on our diet.

DB, aged 44, went on the FastDiet and lost 14 pounds in

a month, but more unexpectedly she also saw big improvements in her lung function. "I have changed nothing else at all, it can only be related to the FastDiet," DB writes. As an experiment she decided to stop doing the diet for a while. "Guess what? My lung function tests have deteriorated significantly. Nothing else has changed. So for me that's proof enough. I am back on the diet tomorrow."

Unfortunately there has not been a lot of scientific research looking at whether intermittent fasting is genuinely helpful for asthma. A few years ago Professor Mark Mattson, of the National Institute on Aging, with Dr. James Johnson, did do a small pilot study of intermittent fasting with ten obese asthmatics (eight women and two men).[20] The overweight asthmatics were put on an alternate-day fasting (ADF) diet for eight weeks. While on this diet they could eat what they wanted one day, then the following day they were asked to cut down to 20 percent of their normal calories. Nine of the ten volunteers managed to stick to the diet for the two months of the trial and actually reported feeling more energetic. They lost an impressive amount of weight, an average of 18 pounds, but what was more surprising is that within a couple of weeks of starting intermittent fasting their asthma symptoms also improved.

Other studies have shown that people who are overweight can experience improvements in their asthma if they lose a lot of weight (at least 13 percent of previous body weight), but the improvements they saw in this study started long before significant weight loss.

It seems something else was going on. The likeliest explanation is that ADF led to a big drop in inflammatory markers. Certain levels of tumor necrosis factor, a measure of chronic inflammation, fell dramatically over the course of the study. Since asthma is largely a disease of inflammation (inflamed airways make breathing harder), then anything that reduces the inflammation is likely to help.

IF and Eczema

Inflammation is also a characteristic feature of eczema (also known as dermatitis), an incredibly common skin condition. Eczema affects around 10 percent of people in Europe and the US. It can be mild, with occasional flare-ups when the skin becomes dry, scaly, and itchy. Or it can be severe, in which case you get weeping, crusting, and bleeding. My daughter had eczema when she was young and we had to battle constantly to stop her scratching. Fortunately, as with many children, the eczema disappeared when she hit her teens, but there is always the risk it will return. We have had a number of people contact us to say their eczema has unexpectedly improved once they started doing the FastDiet.

For example B wrote to say, "For several years I have had eight to ten mildly irritating small eczema patches on my arms and torso. Since I have been doing intermittent fasting, the patches are much, much milder and a few have just disappeared."

Tracy also wrote about the improvements she'd seen: "The total disappearance of my eczema (I used to get quite irritating recurring patches between my fingers) was one of the earliest and happiest side effects of the lifestyle for me. My skin is a million times better in general but the eczema disappearance has made this well worth doing for that reason alone."

Unfortunately I can't find any recent studies on the impact of intermittent fasting on eczema, but if you have eczema and decide to give it a try, do let us know how it goes.

IF and Psoriasis

Psoriasis is an inflammatory skin condition where studies suggest that short periods of fasting may help. Psoriasis can look a lot like eczema. It normally consists of red or silvery, scaly patches that itch. It can appear as just a few patches or cover almost the entire body.

A review article recently published in the *British Journal of Dermatology*[21] asked whether different diets made any difference.

Among the studies was one where twenty patients with arthritis and various skin diseases were put on a two-week modified fast, followed by a three-week vegetarian diet. Not everyone got better, but some patients experienced an improvement. The article concluded that "short-term fasting periods may improve severe symptoms."

Certainly Annette, one of our followers at fastdiet.co.uk, thinks the FastDiet helped her psoriasis. She wrote to us to say: "I used to wake myself up scratching and sore. I started the 5:2 and within days, noticed an improvement. This has continued over the weeks to the point where I can now wear a skirt without tights, unthinkable before I started this diet." Again, more research is badly needed.

Intermittent Fasting: My Personal Journey

As you've read, I started out by trying the four-day fast under Valter Longo's supervision. But despite the improvements in my blood biochemistry and his obvious enthusiasm, I could not imagine doing lengthy fasts on a regular basis for the rest of my life. So, what next? Well, having met Krista Varady and learned all about ADF (alternate-day fasting) I decided to give that a go.

After a short while, however, I realized that it was just too tough physically, socially, and psychologically. It is undoubtedly an effective way to lose weight rapidly and to get powerful changes to your biochemistry, but it was not for me.

So I decided to try eating 600 calories, two days a week. It seemed a reasonable compromise and, more important, doable.

The 5:2 FastDiet is based on a number of different forms of intermittent fasting; it is not based on any one body of research, but is a synthesis.

Before embarking on the diet I decided to get myself properly tested, to see what effects it would have on my body. The following are the tests I did. Most are straight-forward. The blood tests are, with one exception, tests your doctor should be happy to do for you.

Get on the Scale

The first and most obvious thing you will want to do is weigh yourself before embarking on this adventure. Initially, it is best to do this at the same time every day. First thing in the morning is, as I'm sure you know, when you will be at your lightest.

Ideally you should get a weighing machine that measures body fat percentage as well as weight, since what you really want to see is body fat levels fall. The cheaper machines are not fantastically reliable; they tend to underestimate the true figure, giving you a false sense of security. What they are quite good at doing, however, is measuring change. In other words, they might tell you when you start that you are 30 percent body fat when the true figure is closer to 33 percent. But they should be able to tell you when that number begins to fall.

Body Fat

Body fat is measured as a percentage of total weight. The machines you can buy do this by a system called impedance.

There's a small electric current that runs through your body; the machine measures the resistance. It does its estimation based on the fact that muscle and other tissues are better conductors of electricity than fat.

The way to get a truly accurate reading is with a machine called a DXA (formerly DEXA) scanner. It stands for "dual energy X-ray absorptiometry." It is relatively expensive and far more reliable than, say, body mass index. Women tend to have more body fat than men. A man with a body fat percentage of more than 25 percent would be considered overweight. For a woman it would be 30 percent.

Calculate Your BMI

To calculate your body mass index, go to thefastdiet.co.uk where you can track your indices. This will not only do the calculation, but also tell you what it means.

Measure Your Stomach

BMI is useful, but it may not be the best predictor of future health. In a study of more than 45,000 women who were followed for sixteen years, the waist-to-height ratio was a superior predictor of who would develop heart disease.

The reason the waist matters so much is because the worst sort of fat is visceral fat, which collects inside the abdomen. This is the worst sort of distribution because it causes inflammation and puts you at much higher risk of diabetes. You don't need fancy equipment to tell you if you have internal fat. All you need is a tape measure. Male or female, your waist should be less than half your height. Most people underestimate their waist size by about two inches because they rely on pant size. Instead, measure your waist by putting the tape measure around your belly button. Be honest. A definition of optimism is someone who steps on the scale while holding their breath. You are fooling no one.

Blood Tests

You should be able to get standard tests during a routine visit to your doctor.

Fasting Glucose

I chose to measure my fasting glucose because it is a really important measure of fitness even if you are not at risk of diabetes, and it's a predictor of future health. Studies show that even moderately elevated levels of blood glucose are associated with increased risk of heart disease, stroke, and long-term cognitive problems. Ideally I would have had my insulin sensitivity measured, but that test is complex and expensive.

Cholesterol

They measure two types of cholesterol: LDL (low-density lipoprotein) and HDL (high-density lipoprotein). Broadly speaking, LDL carries cholesterol into the wall of your arteries while HDL carries it away. It is good to have a low-ish LDL and a high-ish HDL. One way you can express this is as a percentage of HDL to the sum of HDL plus LDL. Anything over 0.20 (20 percent) is good.

Triglycerides

These are a type of fat that is found in blood; they are one of the ways that the body stores calories. High levels are associated with increased risk of heart disease.

IGF-1

This is an expensive test and not available from every doctor. It is a measure of cell turnover and therefore of cancer risk. It may also be a marker for biological aging. I wanted to find out the effects of 5:2 fasting on my IGF-1. I had discovered that IGF-1 levels drop dramatically in response to a four-day fast, but after a month of normal eating they bounced right back to where they had been before.

My Data

These are the results of the physical measurements I took before starting the FastDiet.

	ME	RECOMMENDED
HEIGHT	5'11" (71 inches)	
WEIGHT	187 lbs.	
BODY MASS INDEX	26.4	19–25
% OF BODY FAT	28%	Less than 25% for men
WAIST SIZE	36 "	Less than half your height
NECK SIZE	17 "	Less than 16½"

I wasn't obese, but both my BMI and my body fat percentage told me that I was overweight. I knew from doing an MRI (magnetic resonance imaging) scan that much of my fat was collected internally, wrapping itself in thick layers around my liver and kidneys, disturbing all sorts of metabolic pathways.

Clearly, the fat wasn't all inside my abdomen. Quite a bit had collected around my neck. This meant that I was snoring. Loudly. Neck size is a powerful predictor[22] of whether you will snore or not. A neck size above 16½ inches for men or 16 inches for women means you are in the danger zone.

	MY RESULTS IN MMOL/L	RECOMMENDED
DIABETES RISK		
FASTING GLUCOSE	7.3	3.9–5.8
HEART DISEASE FACTORS		
TRIGLYCERIDES	1.4	Less than 2.3
HDL CHOLESTEROL	1.8	0.9–1.5
LDL CHOLESTEROL	5.5	Up to 3.0
HEART DISEASE RISK		
HDL % OF TOTAL	23 %	20% and over
CANCER RISK		
SOMATOMEDIN-C (IGF-1)	28.6 nmol/l	11.3–30.9 nmol/l

According to these data, my fasting glucose was worryingly high. I was a diabetic, so far only at the lower end of the range, but clearly heading toward trouble. My LDL was far too high, but I was to some extent protected by the fact that my triglycerides were low and my HDL high. This is not a good picture, though.

My IGF-1 levels were also too high, suggesting rapid turnover of cells and increased cancer risk.

After three months on the FastDiet there were some remarkable changes, as you'll see in these charts.

	ME	RECOMMENDED
HEIGHT	5' 11" (71 inches)	
WEIGHT	168 lbs.	
BODY MASS INDEX	24	19–25
% OF BODY FAT	21%	Less than 25% for men
WAIST SIZE	33"	Less than half your height
NECK SIZE	16"	Less than 16½"

I had lost about 19 pounds, and my BMI and body fat percentage became respectable. I had to go out and buy smaller belts and tighter pants. I could fit into a dinner jacket I hadn't worn for ten years. I had also stopped snoring, which delighted my wife and quite possibly the neighbors. Even better, my blood indicators had improved in a spectacular fashion.

> I had lost about 19 pounds, and my BMI and body fat percentage became respectable. I had to go out and buy smaller belts and tighter pants.

	MY RESULTS IN MMOL/L	RECOMMENDED
DIABETES RISK		
FASTING GLUCOSE	5.0	3.9–5.8
HEART DISEASE FACTORS		
TRIGLYCERIDES	0.6	Less than 2.3
HDL CHOLESTEROL	2.1	0.9–1.5
LDL CHOLESTEROL	3.6	Up to 3.0
HEART DISEASE RISK		
HDL % OF TOTAL	37%	20% and over
CANCER RISK		
SOMATOMEDIN-C (IGF-1)	15.9 nmol/l	11.3–30.9 nmol/l

My wife, Clare, who is a doctor, was astonished. She regularly sees overweight patients with blood chemistry like mine had been and she said that none of the advice she gives them has had anything like the same effect.

For me, the particularly pleasing changes were in my fasting glucose levels and the huge drop in my IGF-1 levels, which matched the changes I had seen after doing a four-day fast.

Clare, however, felt I was losing weight too fast, that I should consolidate for a while. So I decided to go on a 6:1 maintenance program, fasting just one day a week.

What has happened is that my weight has stayed steady at 168 pounds and my blood markers remain in good shape. There are times, around the holiday season, when my weight creeps up, in which case I either go back to 5:2 or have a few days where I just skip lunch.

So What Is the Best Way to Go About Intermittent Fasting?

Let's recap what we've learned. The reason for intermittent fasting—that is, briefly but severely restricting the amount of calories you consume—is that by doing so you are hoping to "fool" your body into thinking it is in a potential famine situation and that it needs to switch from go-go mode to maintenance mode.

The reason our bodies respond to fasting in this way is that we evolved at a time when feast or famine was the norm. Our bodies are designed to respond to stresses and shocks; it makes them healthier, tougher. The scientific term is "hormesis"—what does not kill you makes you stronger.

The benefits of fasting include:

★ Weight loss

★ A reduction of IGF-1, which means that you are reducing your risk of a number of age-related diseases, such as cancer.

★ The switching-on of countless repair genes in response to this stressor.

★ A rest for your pancreas, which will boost the effectiveness of the insulin it produces in response to elevated blood glucose. Increased insulin sensitivity will reduce your risk of obesity, diabetes, heart disease, and cognitive decline.

★ An overall enhancement in your mood and sense of well-being. This may be a consequence of your brain producing increased levels of neurotrophic factor, which will hopefully make you more cheerful and in turn should make fasting more doable.

So much for the science. In the next chapter we discuss what to eat and how to go about starting life as an intermittent faster. How do you put the theory into practice?

CHAPTER TWO

The FastDiet in Practice

THERE ARE, AS WE'VE SEEN, GOOD CLINICAL REASONS to start intermittent fasting. Some, such as its positive effect on blood markers, should be immediately apparent; others will become manifest over time—a cognitive boost, a self-repairing physiology, a greater chance of a longer life. But perhaps the most compelling argument for many is the promise of swift and sustained weight loss while still eating the foods you would eat normally, most of the time. You may view this as incidental to the plan's other forceful health benefits. Or it may be your primary objective. The fact is you will gain both: weight loss *and* better health, two sides of the same coin.

Michael's experience, as illustrated in the previous chapter, should have given you an idea of what to expect. This chapter will reveal more detail: explaining how to start, how it will feel, how to keep going, and how the central tenets of the FastDiet can slip easily into the rhythm of your everyday life. Then it's over to you.

What Does 500/600 Calories Look Like?

Cutting calories to a quarter of your usual daily intake is a significant commitment, so don't be surprised if your first fast day feels like a tough gig. As you progress, the fasts will become second nature and the initial sense of deprivation will diminish, particularly if you remain aware that tomorrow is another day—another day, in fact, when you can eat normally again.

Still, however you cut it, 500 or 600 calories is no picnic; it's not even half a picnic. A large café latte can clock in at over 300 calories, more if you insist on cream, while your usual lunchtime sandwich might easily consume your entire allowance in one huge bite. So be smart. Spend your calories wisely—the menu plans and recipes on pages 145–192 will be useful—but it's also worth having a clear idea of favorite fast-day foods that work for you. Remember to embrace variety: differing textures, punchy flavors, color, and crunch. Together, these will keep your mouth entertained and stop it from frowning at the hardship of it all.

When to Fast

Animal studies, human studies, research, and experiments— as demonstrated in the previous chapter, evidence for the value of fasting is strong. But what happens when you step out of the laboratory and into real life? When and what you eat during your fast is critical to the diet's success. So what's the optimal pattern?

Michael tried several different fasting regimens; the one he settled on as the most sustainable for him is a fast on two nonconsecutive days each week, allowing 600 calories a day, split between breakfast and dinner. For obvious reasons, he named this pattern the 5:2 diet—five days off, two days on, which means that the majority of your time is spent gloriously free from calorie counting. On a fast day, he'll normally have breakfast with his family at around 7:30 a.m. and then aim to have dinner with them at 7:30 p.m., with nothing eaten in between. That way, he gets two twelve-hour periods without food in a twenty-four-hour day, and a happy family at the end of it.

The menu suggestions starting on page 145 are based on this pattern since it is, in his experience, the most straightforward intermittent fasting method.

Mimi, as she describes later in this chapter, found that a slightly different pattern works for her. Sticking to the Fast-Diet's central tenet, she eats 500 calories—but as two meals with an occasional snack (an apple, some carrot sticks) in between, simply because the vast plain between breakfast and supper feels too great, too empty for comfort. There is evidence from trials conducted by Dr. Michelle Harvie[1] and others that this approach will help you lose weight, reduce your risk of breast cancer, and increase insulin sensitivity.

Which approach is better? At this point, given that the science of intermittent fasting is still in its early days, we don't know. On purely theoretical grounds, a longer period without food (Michael's approach) should produce better results. It takes, for example, about 12 hours without food before your body switches into proper fat-burning mode. Valter Longo thinks that longer periods are better. Fasting or not, he almost always skips lunch.

As far as we are aware, there have been no studies, as yet, that attempt to compare the health benefits to people on a fast day of either eating their calories in one go or splitting them into two meals and including the odd snack. When we know more, we will update you.

Professor Mark Mattson at the National Institute on Aging says that by eating your calories as a single meal you might get a modestly greater ketogenic ("fat-burning") effect, compared to three very small meals spread throughout the day. But he also thinks we shouldn't get too hung up about it. "Regardless of whether the 600 calories is consumed as one meal or two or three smaller meals, you will get major health benefits."

We await more trials, but until then it's clear from the many thousands that have tried it, that as long as you stick to the FastDiet, you will enjoy that crucial combination of weight loss, health benefits, and cheerful compliance.

Some people who don't feel hungry at breakfast would rather eat later in the day. That's fine. One of the key researchers in this field starts her day with a late breakfast at around 11:00 a.m. and finishes with supper at 7:00 p.m. Based on the mouse study cited on page 38, it may even be a better approach.

It is, however, only "better" if you actually do it, and a delayed breakfast may not suit some lifestyles, schedules, or bodies. So go with a schedule that suits you. Some fasters, for instance, appreciate the convenience and simplicity of a single 500- or 600-calorie meal, allowing them to ignore food entirely for most of the day. Whatever you choose, it must be your plan, your life. Do it with gusto, but be prepared to experiment within the limits set out by the plan.

What to Eat

It may seem curious to talk about what to eat when you are fasting. But the FastDiet is a modified program, allowing 500 calories for a woman and 600 for a man on any given fast day, making the regimen relatively comfortable and, above all, sustainable over the long term. So, yes, you do get to eat on a fast day. But it matters what you choose.

There are two general principles that should govern what you eat and what you avoid on a fast day. Your aim is to have food that makes you feel satisfied but stays firmly within the 500/600 calorie allowance—and the best options to achieve this are meals that include:

★ foods with a low glycemic index (GF)

★ some protein

The FastDiet is a modified program,
allowing 500 calories for a woman and
600 for a man on any given fast day, making
the regimen relatively comfortable and,
above all, sustainable over the long term.

There have been several studies[2] demonstrating that individuals who eat a higher-protein diet feel fuller for longer (indeed, the main reason people lose weight on diets like Atkins is that they eat less). The trouble with really high protein diets, however, is that people tend to get bored with the food restrictions and give up. There is also evidence that high-protein diets are associated with higher levels of chronic inflammation and IGF-1, which in turn are associated with increased risk of heart disease and cancer.[3]

So the FastDiet does not recommend boycotting carbs entirely, or living permanently on a high-protein diet. However, on a fast day, the combination of proteins and foods with a low glycemic index will be helpful weapons in keeping hunger at bay.

Understanding the Glycemic Index

In earlier chapters, we discussed the importance of blood sugar and insulin. High levels of insulin brought about by high levels of blood sugar will encourage your body to store fat and increase your cancer risk. Another reason not to eat foods that make your blood sugar levels surge, particularly on your fast days, is that when your blood sugar crashes, as it inevitably will, you will start feeling very hungry indeed.

Carbohydrates have the biggest impact on blood sugar, but not all carbs are equal. As habitual dieters will know, one way to discover which carbs cause a big spike and which don't is to look at their glycemic index (GI). Each food gets a score out of 100, with a low score meaning that the particular food does not tend to cause a rapid rise in blood glucose. These are the ones you want.

The size of the sugar spike depends not just on the food itself, but also on how much of it you eat. For example, we tend to eat a lot more potatoes in one sitting than kiwi fruit. So there's also a measure called the glycemic load (GL), which is:

$$GL = \frac{GI \times grams\ of\ carbohydrate}{100}$$

This makes some pretty heroic assumptions about the amount of a particular food you are likely to eat as a portion, but at least it is a guide.

The reason GI and GL are interesting is not just because they are strongly predictive of future health (people on a low GL diet have less risk of diabetes, heart disease, and various cancers), but because there are so many surprises. Who would have imagined that eating a baked potato would have as big an impact on your blood glucose as eating a tablespoon of sugar?

Broadly speaking, a GI over 50 or a GL over 20 is not good, and the lower both figures are, the better. It is worth restating that GI and GL are measures that relate to carbs. GI is not relevant to protein and fats, which is why none of the foods listed have a significant protein or fat content.

Let's take a quick look at breakfast:

BREAKFAST	GI	GL
Oatmeal	50	10
Granola	50	10
Baguette	95	15
Croissant	67	17
Cornflakes	80	20

Source: people.bu.edu/sobieraj/papers/GlycemicIndices.pdf.

You can see why, if you are having a carb breakfast, oatmeal and granola are better options than cornflakes or a croissant.

And what are you going to put on your granola?

	GI	GL
Milk, skim	27	3
Soy milk	44	8

The relatively high GI and GL of soy milk is just one reason to stick with dairy.

What About Protein?

We certainly don't recommend eating protein to the exclusion of all else on a fast day, but you do require an adequate quantity for muscle health, cell maintenance, endocrinal regulation, immunity, and energy. Protein is satiating, too, so it's well worth including it in your calorie quota. It may sound confusing that we recommend protein on your fast day, while elsewhere Michael suggests that too much protein is not good for you. The answer is that while we recommend eating a higher *percentage* of your diet as protein on a fast day, since you are eating significantly fewer calories overall, you are actually consuming relatively modest amounts of protein.

While Valter Longo recommends 0.8g of protein per pound of body weight per day—which would give a 168 pound man around 60g, and a 126 pound woman around 45g—perhaps the simplest method is to stick to recommended governmental guidelines, which allow for a (quite generous) 50g per day.

Go for "good protein." Steamed white fish, for example, is low in saturated fats and rich in minerals. Choose skinless chicken over red meat; try low-fat dairy products over endless lattes; include shrimp, tuna, and tofu or other plant-based proteins. Nuts, seeds, and legumes (beans, peas, and lentils) are full of fiber and act as bulking agents on a hungry day. Nuts, though high in calories (depending, of course, on how much you eat), are generally low GI and brilliantly satiating. They are fatty, too, so you might imagine they are "bad for you," yet the evidence is that nut consumers have lower rates of heart disease and diabetes than nut abstainers.[4]

Eggs, meanwhile, are low in saturated fat and full of nutritional value; they won't adversely affect your cholesterol levels and they score around 85 calories each (that's for a medium/large egg). What's more, research suggests that individuals who consume egg protein for breakfast are more likely to feel full during the day than those whose breakfasts contain wheat protein.[5] So an egg-based breakfast on a fast day makes perfect sense. Two eggs plus a 1¾-ounce serving of smoked salmon, for example, clock in at a sensible 250 calories. Poaching or boiling an egg avoids the addition of careless calories.

For more suggestions about foods to keep you full on a fast day, and the benefits certain choices will bring, turn to page 190.

How to Fit Fasting into Your Life

When to Start?

If you do not have an underlying medical condition, and if you are not an individual for whom fasting is not advised (see pages 132–133), then there really is no time like the present. Ask yourself: if not now, when? You may prefer to await a doctor's advice. You may choose to prepare yourself—to talk yourself down from a lifelong habit of overeating, to clear out the fridge, to eat the last cookie in the jar (there are plenty of tips for preparation on pages 81–89). Or you may want to get on with it and start to see visible progress within a couple of weeks. Do, however, begin on a day when you feel strong, purposeful, calm, and committed. Do tell friends and family that you're starting the FastDiet; once you make a public commitment, you are much more likely to stick with it. Avoid holidays, vacations, and days when you've got to attend a fancy business lunch complete with bread basket, cheese course, and four types of dessert. Recognize, too, that a busy day will help your fast time fly, while a lazy one generally goes as slow as molasses.

Once you've deliberated and designated a day to debut, get your mind in gear. Record your details—weight, BMI, waist, target weight—in a diary before you start, and be ready to note your progress, knowing that dieters who keep an honest account of what they eat and drink are more likely to lose the pounds and keep them off. Then . . . take a deep breath and relax. Better yet, shrug. It's no big deal, just a brief break from eating: you have nothing to lose but weight.

How Tough Will It Be?

If it has been a while since you have experienced hunger, even the slightest hint, you'll probably find that eating no more than 500 or 600 calories in a day is a mild challenge, at least initially. Intermittent fasters do report that the process becomes significantly easier with time, particularly as they witness results in the mirror and on the scale. Though your first fast day may be challenging, it's equally possible that it will speed by, buoyed along by the novelty of the process; a fast day on a wet Wednesday in week three may feel more of a slog. Your mission is to complete it, knowing that although you are saying no to chocolate today, you will be eating normally tomorrow. That is the joy of the FastDiet and what makes it so different from other weight-loss plans.

Although you are saying no to chocolate today, you will be eating normally tomorrow. That is the joy of the FastDiet and what makes it so different from other weight-loss plans.

How to Win the Hunger Games

There is no reason to be alarmed by benign, occasional, short-term hunger. Given base-level good health, you will not perish. You won't collapse in a heap and need to be rescued by the cat. Your body is designed to go without food for longish periods, even if it has lost the skill through years of grazing, picking, and snacking. Research has found that modern humans tend to mistake a whole range of emotions for hunger.[6] We eat when we're bored, when we're thirsty, when we're around food (when aren't we?), when we're with company, or simply when the clock happens to tell us it's time for food. Most of us eat, too, just because it feels good.

This "hedonic eating" can readily overcome the body's natural satiety signals: You'll recognize it if you eat for reasons other than hunger. The kicker might be social (shared lunches, communal eating, everyone at the table agreeing to order dessert); it may be environmental (scheduled mealtimes, which persuade you that you're hungry even when you're not; the arrival of bread at the beginning of a meal), or emotional (comfort eating, the popcorn that makes a movie more of a treat, the tub of ice cream demolished when you're feeling blue).

While you should try to resist hedonic eating on a fast day, you can bask in the knowledge that, if you please, you can give in to a little temptation the following day.

There's no need to panic about any of this. Simply note that the human brain is adept at persuading us that we're hungry in almost all situations: when faced with feelings of deprivation or withdrawal or disappointment; when angry, sad, happy, neutral; when subjected to advertising, social imperatives, sensory stimulation, reward, habit, the smell of freshly brewed coffee or bread baking or bacon cooking in a café up the road. Recognize now that these are often learned reactions to external cues, most of them designed to part you from your cash. On a fast day, if you are still processing your last meal, it's highly unlikely that what you are experiencing is true hunger ("total transit time," should you be interested in such things, can take up to two days, depending on your gender, your metabolism, and what you've eaten).

While hunger pangs can be aggressive and disagreeable, in practice they are more fluid and controllable than you might think. You're unlikely to be troubled at all by hunger until well into a fast day. What's more, a pang will pass. Fasters report that the feeling of perceived hunger comes in waves, not in an ever-growing wall of gnawing belly noise. It's a symphony of differentiated movements, not a steady, fearful crescendo. Treat a tummy rumble as a good sign, a healthy messenger.

Remember, too, that hunger does not build over a twenty-four-hour period, so don't feel trapped in the feeling at any given moment. Wait a while. You have absolute power to conquer feelings of hunger, simply by steering your mind, riding the wave, choosing to do something else—take a walk, phone a friend, drink tea, go for a run, take a shower. . . . After a few weeks' practicing intermittent fasting, people generally report that their sense of hunger is diminished.

The main struggle with doing the FastDiet or any form of fasting is the first few weeks while your body and mind adjust to new habits, new ways of eating. The good news is that most people find they soon adapt. In fact many people have contacted us to say that it is unexpectedly easy.

The important thing is to have a strategy that suits you. Try to decipher your hunger. Are you really hungry? Or are you overriding your brain's satiety message? Even posing the question can be enough to still the urge. There are practical ways to circumvent the feeling too: the real trick is to eat foods that keep you feeling fuller longer. This means some protein. This means slow-burn, low-GI fuel. This means bulk from plants.

Compliance and Sustainability: Finding a Sensible Eating Pattern that Works for You

Most diets don't work. You know that already. Indeed, when a team of psychologists at UCLA conducted an analysis of thirty-one long-term diet trials back in 2007, they concluded that "several studies indicate that dieting is a consistent predictor of future weight gain. . . . We asked what evidence is there that dieting works in the long term, and found that the evidence shows the opposite." Their analysis found that while dieters on conventional diets do lose pounds in the early months, the vast majority return to their original weight within five years, while "at least a third end up heavier than when they embarked on the project."[7] The standard approach clearly doesn't work.

In order to be effective, then, any method must be rational, sustainable, flexible, and feasible over the long haul. Adherence, not weight loss per se, is the key, so your goals must be realistic and the program practical. It must fit into your life as it is, not the life of your dreams. It needs to go on vacation with you, it needs to visit friends, get you through a boring (or challenging) day at the office, and cope with Christmas. To work at all, any weight-loss strategy has to be tolerable, organic, and innate, not some spurious add-on that makes you feel awkward and self-conscious, the dietary equivalent of uncomfortable shoes.

While the long-term experience of intermittent fasters is still under investigation, people who have tried it comment on how easily it fits into everyday life. They still get variety from food (anyone who's ever tried to lose weight on only grapefruit or cabbage soup will know how vital this is). They still get rewards from food. They still get a life. There is no drama, no desperate dieting, no self-flagellation. No sweat.

Tomorrow Is Another Day: The FastDiet's Appeal

Perhaps the most reassuring and game-changing part of the FastDiet is that it doesn't last forever. Unlike deprivation diets that have failed you before, on this plan tomorrow will always be different. Easier. There may be pancakes for breakfast, or lunch with friends, wine with supper, apple pie with ice cream. This on/off switch is critical. It means that on a fast day, though you're eating a quarter of your usual calorie intake, tomorrow you can eat as you please. There's boundless psychological comfort in the fact that your fasting will only ever be a short stay, a brief break from food.

When you're not fasting, ignore fasting—it doesn't own you, it doesn't define you. You're not even doing it most of the time. Unlike full-time fad diets, you'll still get pleasure from food, you'll still have treats, you'll engage in the regular, routine, food-related events of your normal life. There are no special shakes, bars, rules, points, affectations, or idiosyncrasies. No saying "no" all the time. For this reason, you won't feel serially deprived, which—as anyone who has embarked on the grinding chore of long-term every-

> Unlike full-time fad diets, you'll still get pleasure from food, you'll still have treats, you'll engage in the regular, routine, food-related events of your normal life.

day dieting knows—is precisely why conventional diet plans fail.

The key, then, is to recognize, through patience and the exercise of will, that you can make it through to breakfast tomorrow. Bear in mind that fasting subjects regularly report that the food with which they "break their fast" tastes glorious. Flavors sing. Mouthfuls dance. If you've ever felt a lazy disregard for the food you consume without thinking, then things are about to change. There's nothing like a bit of delayed gratification to make things taste good.

Flexibility: Your Key to Success

Your body is not my body. Mine is not yours. So it's worth carving out your plan according to your needs, the shape of your day, your family, your commitments, your preferences. None of us live cookie-cutter lives, and no single diet plan fits all. Everyone has quirks and qualifiers. That's why there are no absolute commandments here, just suggestions. You may choose to fast in a particular way, on a particular day. You may like to eat once, or twice, first thing or last. You may like beets or fennel or blueberries. Some individuals prefer to be told exactly what to eat and when; others like a more informal approach. That's fine. It's enough to simply stick to the basic method—500 or 600 calories a day, with as long a window without food as possible, twice a week—and you'll gain the plan's multiple benefits. In time, there's little need for assiduous calorie counting; you'll know what a fast day means and how to make it suit you. You can, however, stack the odds in your favor . . . by changing your mind.

Mind and Motivation: How to Master Habit, Temptation, and Willpower

Since we first published *The FastDiet* back in 2013, one of the topics that has regularly come up in the chat rooms and on our website—and in the street or in the coffee line—is how to deal with ingrained habits around food. Fasting, even for relatively short periods, even with calories coming in, quite obviously requires not only self-motivation, but a generous degree of self-control.

On average, we make 227 food-related decisions every day (most people, when questioned, wildly underestimate the number and guess that it's about 14).[8] That's plenty of choice, and plenty of opportunities to collapse into the embrace of the nearest gingerbread man. Over the last two years, we've compiled some strategies to help you arm yourself instead. The basic message is to notice *in advance* the traps and the trip wires to come. These will be personal to you—your very own map of habits and routines that may frustrate a fast day. A few tips should help you navigate the terrain ahead.

★ **Know your triggers.** When you experience a compulsion to eat too much, or to break a fast, it's time to face it head-on. You are a rational being and you are making a specific, time-sensitive decision to eat that sandwich or pour that glass of wine. You really do have the power to choose, at each incremental, individual moment. Once you appreciate this power, it is possible to overcome the cognitive bias that leads to impulsive snacking and compulsive eating—certainly for long enough to get you through a fast day. Recognize—before it happens—when your self-control is likely to dissolve. Try to install a behavior—not forever, just for that precise moment—that alters your established route. This is called "deliberate practice"; it takes grit, determination, and a certain amount of self-awareness. If, for instance, you're always ravenous when you get home from work on a fast day, make sure there's an apple stashed in your bag to eat en route (and include it in your calorie count for that day). Have business lunches in the office or in a park, not in a restaurant where they serve the world's best tiramisu. If you're prone to a late-night forage in the fridge, run a bath instead.

★ **Understand that temptation, when it comes, is fleeting.** Prepare to distract yourself, if only for five minutes—count backward, concentrate on your breathing, sing, run upstairs to make the bed, fetch a glass of water, stroll across the office to speak to a friend. Small actions? Yes, but powerful enough for that particular and distinct moment of craving to pass.

★ **Employ the "Proximity Principle" and put temptation out of reach.** As one study (using Hershey's Kisses) showed, having food conveniently close at hand makes you eat a great deal more of it.[9] On a fast day, don't give yourself the choice of whether to eat the cookies or not; hide the cookies. Better yet, don't buy the cookies. Buy more fresh vegetables and have them handy instead.

★ **Ensure that your goal outweighs your temptation.** This may seem obvious (otherwise, you'd never get going). But you need reminding, at the very instant of seduction, that you're fasting for very good reasons: for weight loss, better health, longer life. Perhaps try site-specific aversion therapy. If necessary, tape a picture of yourself—the selfie you'd never post on Facebook, the holiday snap that made you embark on the FastDiet in the first place—to the fridge door.

★ **Exercise willpower.** I mean really "exercise" it. In her book *The Willpower Instinct*, Stanford psychologist Kelly McGonigal suggests that self-control shouldn't be seen as a virtue, but as a muscle: it gets tired from use, but regular exercise makes it stronger. This is great news: it means (as we know from experience on the FastDiet) that the going gets easier if we persevere.

The Maintenance Model

Once you've reached your target weight or just a shade below (allowing room for flexibility and a generous slice of birthday cake), you may consider adopting the Maintenance Model. This is an adjustment to fasting on just one day each week—going from 5:2 to 6:1—in order to remain in a holding pattern at your desired weight but still reap the benefits of occasional fasting. Naturally, one day a week may offer fewer health benefits in the long run than two; but it does fit neatly into your life, particularly if you are not intent on achieving any further weight loss. Equally, if the beach beckons or there's a wedding on the calendar or you've woken up on the day after Christmas haunted by that fourth roast potato, step it back up. You're in charge.

What to Expect

The first thing you can expect from adopting the FastDiet, of course, is to lose weight—some weeks more, some weeks less; some weeks finding yourself stuck at a disappointing plateau, other weeks making swifter progress. As a basic guide, you might anticipate a loss of around 1 to 2 pounds a week. This will not, of course, be all fat. Some will be water, and some the digested food in your system. You should, however, lose around ten pounds of fat over a ten-week period, which beats a typical low-calorie diet. Crucially, you can expect to maintain your weight loss over time.

More important than what you'll lose, though, is what you're set to gain.

How Your Anatomy Will Change

Over a period of weeks, you can expect your BMI, body fat percentage, and waist measurement to drop and your lean muscle mass to increase. Your cholesterol count, blood glucose, and IGF-1 levels may improve. This is the path to greater health and extended life. You are already dodging your unwritten future. Right now, though, the palpable changes will start to show up in the mirror as your body becomes leaner and lighter.

As the weeks progress, you'll find that intermittent fasting has potent secondary effects, too.

> Over a period of weeks, you can expect your BMI, body fat percentage, and waist measurement to drop and your lean muscle mass to increase. Your cholesterol count, blood glucose, and IGF-1 levels may improve.

Alongside the obvious weight loss and health benefits stored up for the future, there are more subtle consequences, perks, and bonuses that can come into play.

How Your Appetite Will Change

Expect your food preferences to adapt; pretty soon, you'll start to choose healthy foods by default, not by design. You will begin to understand hunger, to negotiate and manage it, knowing how it feels to be properly hungry. You'll also recognize the sensation of being pleasantly full, not groaning like an immovable sofa. Satiated, not stuffed. The upshot? No more "food hangovers," improved digestion, more bounce.

After six months of intermittent fasting, interesting things should happen to your eating habits. You may find that you eat half the meat you once did—not as a conscious move, but a natural one born of what you desire rather than what you decide or believe. You're likely to consume more vegetables. Many intermittent fasters instinctively retreat from bread (and, by association, butter), while stodgy "comfort" foods seem less appealing and refined sugars aren't nearly as tempting as they once were.

Of course, you don't need to dwell actively on any of this. If you are like me, then one day soon, you'll arrive at a place where you say no to the cheesecake because you don't want it, not because you are denying yourself a treat. This is the baseline power of intermittent fasting: it encourages you to recheck your diet. And that's your long-haul ticket to health.

How Your Attitude Will Change

So yes, you'll start to lose bad habits around food. But if you continue to fast—and eat—with awareness, all kinds of other changes should occur, some of them unlikely and unexpected. You may, for instance, discover that you've been suffering from "portion distortion" for years, thinking that the food piled on your plate is the quantity you really need and want. With time, you'll probably discover that you've been overdoing it. Muffins will start to look vast as they sit, fat and moist, under glass domes in the coffee shops. A large bag of chips becomes a monstrous prospect. You may go from venti to grande to only wanting half a cup, no sugar, no cream.

Soon you'll come to recognize the truth about how you've been eating and the wordless fibs you've told yourself for years. This is as much a part of the recalibrating process as anything else; you've changed your mind. Occasional fasting will train you in the art of "restrained eating"; at the end of the day, this is the goal. It's all part of the long game of behavioral change that means that the FastDiet will ultimately become neither a fast nor a diet, but a way of life. After a while, you'll have cultivated a new approach to eating—thoughtful, rational, responsible—without even knowing you're doing it.

Intermittent fasters also report a boost to their energy, together with an amplified sense of emotional well-being. Some talk of a "glow"—the result, perhaps, of winning the battle for self-control, or from the smaller clothes and the compliments, or from something going on at a metabolic level that governs our moods. We may not yet know precisely why, but whatever it is, it feels good. Far better than cake. As one online devotee says, "Overall, fasting just seems right. It's like a reset button for your entire body." [10]

More subtly still, many fasters acknowledge a sense of relief as their fast days no longer revolve around food. Embrace it. There's a certain liberty here, if you allow it to materialize. You may find, as we have, that you start to look forward to your fasts: a time to regroup and give feeding a rest.

The FastDiet in Reality:
Tales, Tips, and Troubleshooting

How Men Fast:
Michael's Experience

A lot of men have contacted me to let me know how much weight they have lost and also how surprised and delighted they are that intermittent fasting turns out to be so easy. They like its simplicity, the fact that you don't have to give things up or try to remember complicated recipes. I also think they rather like the challenge.

One of the things that men seem to like particularly about fasting is that they can fit it into their lives with minimal hassle. It doesn't stop them working, traveling, socializing, or exercising. In fact, some find it fuels performance (see pages 129–130 for more on fasting and exercise).

In one Belgian study, men asked to eat a high-fat diet and exercise before breakfast on an empty stomach put on far less weight than a similar group of men on an identical diet who exercised after breakfast.[11] This study lends support to the claim that eating in a fasted state makes the body burn a greater percentage of fat for fuel. At least it does if you are a man.

For me, a fast day now follows a familiar routine. I start with a protein-rich breakfast, normally scrambled eggs or a dish of cottage cheese. I drink several cups of black coffee and tea during the day, work happily through lunch, and rarely feel any hunger pangs until well into the late afternoon. When they happen, I simply ignore them or go for a brief stroll until they pass.

In the evening I have a bit of meat or fish and piles of steamed vegetables. Having abstained since breakfast, I find them particularly delicious. I never have problems getting to sleep and most days wake up the next morning feeling no more peckish than normal.

How Women Fast: Mimi's Experience

While most men I know respond well to numbers and targets (with associated gadgets, if at all possible), I've found that women tend to take a more holistic approach to fasting. As with much in life, we like to examine how it feels, knowing that our bodies are unique and will respond to any given stimulation in their own sweet way. We respond to shared stories and the support of friends. And, sometimes, we need a snack.

Personally, for instance, I like to consume my fast-day calories in two lots—one early, one late—bookending the day with my allowance and aiming for a longish gap in between to maximize the prospect of health gains and weight loss. But I do sometimes need a little something to keep me going in between. A fast-day breakfast is usually a low-sugar muesli, perhaps including some fresh strawberries and almonds, with 1% or 2% milk; there'll be an apple for lunch—hardly a feast, I know, but just enough to make a difference to the day. Then, supper at 7-ish: a substantial, interesting salad with heaps of leaves and some lean protein—perhaps smoked salmon or tuna or hummus. Throughout the day, I drink mineral water with a squeeze of lime, tons of herbal tea, and plenty of black coffee. They just help the day tick by.

In my first four months on the FastDiet, I lost 13.2 pounds, and my BMI went from 21.4 to 19.4. If you're struggling with bigger numbers than these, take strength from the fact that heavier subjects respond brilliantly to intermittent fasting, and the positive effects should be apparent in a relatively short time. These days, one fast a week (on Mondays) seems to suffice and keep me at a stable, happy weight.

Many women I encounter are well versed in dieting

techniques (years of practice), and I've found a couple of tips that come in handy on a fast day. I recommend, for instance, eating in small mouthfuls, chewing slowly, and concentrating when eating. If you're getting only 500 calories, it makes sense to notice them as they go in.

Like many intermittent fasters, I have found that hunger is simply not an issue. For whatever reason—and one wonders whether it suits the food industry—we have developed a fear of hunger, fretting about low blood sugar and whatnot. On the whole, for me, a day with little food feels emancipated rather than restrictive. That said, there are ups and downs: some days skip by like a pebble on water; other days, I feel like I'm sinking, not swimming, perhaps because emotions or hormones or simply the tricky business of life have kicked in. See how you feel, and always give in gracefully if that particular day is not your day to fast.

A Dozen Ways to Make the FastDiet Work for You

1. **Know your weight, your BMI, and your waist size from the get-go.** As we mentioned earlier, waist measurement is a simple and important gauge of internal fat and a powerful predictor of future health. BMI is your weight (in pounds) divided by your height (in inches) squared, multiplied by a conversion factor of 703 (or you can just let a BMI website do the calculation); it may sound like

palaver, and an abstract one at that, but it's the best tool we have to plot a path to healthy weight loss. Do note that a BMI score takes no account of body type, age, or ethnicity, and so should be greeted with informed caution. Still, if you need a number, this is a useful one.

Weigh yourself regularly but not obsessively. Once or twice a week should suffice. The mornings after fast days are best if you like to see falling figures. You may discover that your weight is significantly different from day to day. This discrepancy may well be due to the additional weight of food in your system rather than from changes in your fat mass from one day to the next. You may prefer to take an average over several days to arrive at a reasonable figure for any weight loss. But don't overdo it; try not to make weighing— yourself or your calories—a chore.

2. **Chart your progress.** If you are someone who enjoys structure and clarity, you may want to monitor your progress (you'll find a helpful progress tracker on our website). Have a target in mind. Where do you want to be, and when? Be realistic: precipitous weight loss is not advised, so allow yourself time. Make a plan. Write it down. Aim to be specific: if you want to lose weight, there is a psychological advantage in setting a defined goal for how much weight you want to

lose (10 pounds?) and by when (March 15 for your sister's wedding?).

Plenty of people recommend keeping a diet diary. Dieters who write daily notes are known to be more successful at losing weight than those who don't, with one study[12] finding that it can double weight loss as part of a managed program. Logging consumption seems to heighten awareness; the simple act of quantifying incoming food (and, don't forget, drink) seems to strengthen your hand. Alongside the numbers and food notes, consider adding your fast day experiences; try to note three good things that happen each day. It's a feel-good message that you can refer to as time goes by. It helps too, in psychologists' jargon, to "reframe the motivator." Rather than thinking "Arrgh, I don't want to be fat," focus on "I'd like to be slimmer, healthier, and full of energy." Consider what you want, frame it positively, write it down, and read it every day.

3. **Find a fast friend.** You need very few accoutrements to make this a success, but a supportive friend may well be one of them. Once you're on the FastDiet, tell people about it; you may find that they join in, and you'll develop a network of common experience. Since the plan appeals to men and women equally, couples report that they find it more manageable to do it together.

That way you get mutual support, camaraderie, joint commitment, and shared anecdotes; besides, mealtimes are made infinitely easier if you're eating with someone who understands the rudiments of the plot. There are plenty of threads on online chat rooms and forums, which are great sources of support and information. Over the past two years, the 5:2 conversation has been evolving and growing online. To tune in to the discussion, and to discover countless tips to make the FastDiet work for you, go to www.thefastdiet.co.uk. Or investigate the many Facebook groups—ours is at www.facebook.com/thefastdiet.co.uk. It's remarkable how reassuring it is to know that you're not alone.

4. **Prep your fast-day food in advance** so that you don't go foraging and come across a leftover sausage lurking irresistibly in the fridge. Shop and cook on nonfast days, so as not to taunt yourself with unnecessary temptation. Keep it simple, aiming for flavor without effort. (For simple, sustaining recipe ideas, see pages 169–185.) Before you embark on the FastDiet, clear the house of junk food. It will only croon and coo at you from the cupboard, making your fast day harder than it needs to be. Eliminate illicit food stashes; empty your snack drawer at work. And don't forget to check calorie labels for portion size. When the cereal box says "a 30g serving," weigh it out. Go on. Be amazed. Then

be honest. Since your calorie count on a fast day is necessarily fixed and limited, it's important not to be blinkered about how much is actually going in. You'll find a quick calorie counter on pages 205–210.

5. **Wait before you eat.** Try to resist for at least ten minutes, fifteen if you can, to see if the hunger subsides (as it naturally tends to do). The idea here is to put food in its place. It's only food. Once you start to think about food in a rational and realistic way, you'll discover that you can modify your behavior around it. You can even push it aside. You may discover, as many fasters attest, that you develop a keen sensitivity to your own appetite, hunger, satiety, digestion, metabolism. They will change from day to day. Stay quiet, and you can begin to feel these subtle, visceral things.

On fast days, eat with awareness, allowing yourself to fully absorb the fact that you're eating (not as daft as it sounds, particularly if you have ever sat in a traffic jam popping M&M's). Similarly, on off-duty days, stay gently alert. Eat until you're satisfied, not until you're full (this will come naturally after a few weeks' practice). Work out what the concept of "fullness" means for you— we are all different, and it changes over time.

6. **Stay busy.** "We humans are always looking for things to do between meals," said singer-songwriter

Leonard Cohen. Yes, and look where it's got us.

So fill your day, not your face. As fasting advocate Brad Pilon has noted, "No one's hungry in the first few seconds of a skydive." Engage in things other than food—not necessarily skydiving, but anything that appeals to you. Distraction is your best defense against the dark arts of the food industry, which has stationed doughnuts on every street corner and nachos at every turn. And remember, if you absolutely must have that doughnut, it will still be there tomorrow.

7. **Experiment.** The key, as we've established, is to find a plan that works for you, which means you may need to experiment a little until you find your best fit for a sustainable, lifelong plan, not merely a short-lived practice. Rather than think of 5:2 as a "diet," which in its modern usage is larded with quick-fix connotations, perhaps begin to see it as stemming from the classical Greek "diaita." This roughly translates as a "manner of living." A way of life. So, be playful. Customize.

8. **Don't be afraid to think about food you like.** A psychological mechanism called habituation—in which the more people have of something, the less value they attach to it—means that doing the opposite and trying to suppress thoughts of food is probably a flawed strategy.[13] The critical thought

process here is to treat food as a friend, not a foe. Food is not magical, supernatural, or dangerous. Don't demonize it; normalize it. It's only food. Try not to associate fasting with discomfort; be gentle to cultivate the changes you desire; don't dwell on the downside if, say, a fast day is broken. Move on.

9. **Stay hydrated.** Find no-calorie drinks you like, and then drink them in quantity. Some swear by herbal tea, others prefer mineral water with bubbles to dance on the tongue, though tap water will do just as well. Plenty of our hydration comes through the food we eat, so fasters may need to compensate with additional drinks beyond their routine intake (check your urine; it should be plentiful and pale). While there's no scientific rationale for drinking the recommended eight glasses of water a day, there is good reason to keep the liquids coming in. A dry mouth is the last sign of dehydration, not the first, so act before your body complains, recognizing too that a glass of water is a quick way to hush an empty belly, at least temporarily. It will also stop you from mistaking thirst for hunger.

10. **Don't count on weight loss on any given day**. If you have a week when the scale doesn't seem to shift, dwell instead upon the health benefits you will certainly be accruing even if you haven't seen your numbers drop. Remember why you're doing this: not

just the smaller jeans, but the long-term advantages: the widely accepted disease-busting, brain-boosting, life-lengthening benefits of intermittent fasting. Think of it as a pension plan for your body. So keep your perspective: don't be disheartened if you "plateau" in any given week; weight loss is your bonus, not your sole objective.

11. **Be sensible, exercise caution, and if it feels wrong, stop**. It's vital that this strategy should be practiced in a way that's flexible and forgiving. If you're concerned about any aspect of intermittent fasting, see your doctor. Remember, too, that it's okay to break the rules if you need to. It's not a race to the finish, so be kind and make it fun.

12. **Congratulate yourself**. Every completed fast day means potential weight loss and quantifiable health gain. You're already winning. So? Say so. A study from the University of Chicago[14] reveals how positive feedback on new habits will increase the likelihood of success. Don't be afraid to grandstand your achievements. Website forums make an ideal platform for a bit of back-patting— go to www.thefastdiet.co.uk to see tons of support and praise in action. Plenty of people on our site say that this is often enough to get them through a tricky patch.

Q & A

"Fasting is a fiery weapon. It has its own science. No one, as far as I'm aware, has a perfect knowledge of it."

—Gandhi

Which days should I choose to fast?

It really doesn't matter. It's your life, and you'll know which days will suit you best. Monday is an obvious choice for many, perhaps because it is more manageable, psychologically and practically, to gear yourself up at the beginning of a new week, particularly if it follows a sociable weekend. For that reason, fasters might choose to avoid Saturdays and Sundays, when family lunches and brunches, dinner dates and parties make calorie-cutting a chore. Thursday would then make a sensible second fasting day, chiming, if such things appeal to you, with the teachings of the Prophet Muhammad, who is understood to have fasted on the second and fifth days of the week. But be flexible; don't force yourself to fast when it feels wrong. If you're particularly stressed, off-kilter, tired, or peevish on a day that you have designated a fast, try again another day. Adapt. This is not about one-size-fits-all rules; it's about finding a realistic pattern that works for you. Do, however, aim for a pattern. That way, over time your fasts will become familiar, a low-key habit you accept and embrace. You may adapt your fasts as your life—and your body—change shape. But don't drop too many fast days; there is a danger that you'll slide back into old habits. Be kind. But be tough.

When should I eat?

Go with a timetable that suits you. As we've seen, some fasters appreciate the convenience and simplicity of a single 500/600-calorie evening meal, allowing them to ignore food entirely for most of the day; some people say they actually feel hungrier during the day if they have breakfast. Having just one meal, as late in the day as possible, will clearly intensify the fast—allowing your body a longer period in which to enter a fasted state.

Others prefer to eat breakfast and then avoid food for a "fasting window" of around twelve hours until supper. Since it is the fasted state that is so beneficial to us, eating lots of small meals is likely to reduce the benefits, particularly if you graze on carbohydrates. Remember that over time, as you get used to the diet, your body should acclimate to periods of fasting; so keep your personal pattern flexible and adjust to a more lengthy fasting window when you feel able. Stay alert and tweak the regimen to suit your needs.

Does it have to be for twenty-four hours?

Fasting for a "day" is practical, coherent, and unambiguous, all of which will promise a greater chance of success. It is, however, only the most convenient way of organizing a fast. There's nothing magical about it. To save on bother, stick to the idea of a "fast day," and remind yourself that you'll be asleep for nearly a third of it.

In reality, of course, a "fast day," with its 500/600-calorie allowance, lasts up to thirty-six hours: if you finish your last full evening meal at 7:30 p.m. on Sunday, and Monday is your fast day, you will eat normally again on Tuesday morning at around 7:30 a.m. That is thirty-six hours. But don't get too particular about the numbers; the crux is that during a calendar "day," your calorie consumption is slashed to a quarter of your usual intake.

Should I fast on consecutive days?

Some people like to fast on consecutive days, others prefer to have at least one day off between fast days. There are pros and cons.

If you do back-to-back fasts, your body will spend longer in the fasted state, which is, generally speaking, a good thing. Many people also like the pattern of, say, fasting on a Monday and Tuesday, ensuring that they get their two days over and done with, allowing them to relax for the rest of the week.

The danger, however, of fasting for two days in a row is that you may start to feel resentful, bored, and beleaguered—precisely the feelings that wreck the best-made diet intentions.

Michael tried the consecutive system and found it too challenging to be sustainable over time, so he switched to the split version—fasting on Mondays and Thursdays. The weight loss and the improvements in glucose, cholesterol, and IGF-1 that he saw are all based on this nonconsecutive, two-day pattern.

How much weight will I lose?

This will depend on your metabolism, your individual body type, your starting weight, your level of activity, how effectively and honestly you fast, and how much you eat and drink on your nonfast days. Be judicious: abrupt weight loss is not advised and shouldn't be your aim: with rapid weight loss you will be losing a lot of muscle, which is not your goal.

In the Dublin study Michael mentioned earlier, which involved a combination of 5:2 and three short bursts of HIT a week, there was an average weight loss of 10 pounds over twelve weeks, all of it fat. In Dr. Krista Varady's studies, where the subjects did the more intense alternate-day fasting, they lost an average of between 6 and 11 pounds, almost all fat. Those who also did forty minutes of exercise three times a week lost an average of 14 pounds.

In most intermittent fasting studies, there is impressive fat loss around the gut, with 2 to 3 inches being lost around the waist.

What can I do if I'm not losing weight?

★ Be patient. Some people will take longer than others to start losing weight. Remember to measure yourself around the waist, as what you really want to lose is fat.

★ Be realistic. Although some people lose a lot of weight straight off, the average is more likely to be 1 to 2 pounds a week. It will happen.

★ Watch what you are eating on your nonfast days. The FastDiet is not a free ticket to the all-u-can-eat buffet on the days when you're not fasting. Stay aware. Be sensible. Avoid bingeing. Yes, have treats, but make them a treat in the old-fashioned sense. These days, "treats" are almost a food group in their own right; return them to their rightful place as occasional pleasures.

★ Keep a diary of everything you eat and drink for a week. Then look at the calorie content. Some foods may leap out. I was horrified to discover a muffin can be anywhere between 300 and 600 calories. And just because it says "low fat" on the packet, it doesn't mean that it is low calorie. Some "low-fat" foods (like muffins . . .) can contain more calories than the normal variety.

★ Look at the calories you are getting from drinks. Juices, lattes, alcohol, fizzy drinks, smoothies—they all contain a glut of calories. If you can graduate to drinking more water and sugar-free tea/coffee, that will help. Bear in mind that calories in drinks do not satiate: eat three apples and they will fill you up; drinking three apples in the form of a juice won't.

★ Moving more will certainly help. Michael always takes the stairs, even up seven flights. Get a pedometer and try to build up to doing 10,000 steps a day (most people do less than 5,000). Exercise plus fasting will really help you keep the weight off. For more on incorporating exercise, see page 329–331.

★ Try adding another fast day; go for a 4:3 pattern (four days normal eating, three days of reduced calories). Or you might consider alternate-day fasting, particularly ADF plus exercise. In the study quoted above, people doing ADF plus exercise lost, on average, 14 pounds in twelve weeks.

Will I go into starvation mode?

The short answer is an emphatic "no." This is one of the great dieting myths—the fear that if you cut your calories for even a day, then your metabolic rate will slow right down as your body tries to conserve its fat stores. This starvation mode myth seems to be based on the Minnesota starvation experiment, a study carried out during World War II. In this experiment, young volunteers lived on extremely low calorie diets for up to six months. The purpose of the study was to help scientists understand how to treat victims of mass starvation in Europe.

After prolonged starvation, when their body fat had fallen to less than 10 percent, there was a drop in body temperature and heart rate, suggesting that their basal metabolic rate (the energy burned by your body when you are at rest) had fallen. This, however, was an extreme situation.

A more recent experiment on the effects of short-term calorie restriction produced very different results. In this study, from the University of Vienna,[15] they took eleven healthy volunteers and asked them to live on nothing but water for eighty-four hours (in other words, a four-day fast). The researchers then measured the volunteers' metabolic rate at the end of each day. They found that their metabolic rates actually went up; after four days without food, they were 12 percent higher than at the beginning.

One reason for this may have been that they measured a

significant rise in blood levels of a catecholamine called noradrenaline, which is known to burn fat. If they had continued the experiment, the volunteers' metabolic rates would eventually have fallen, not least because they would have begun to lose significant amounts of weight. But, certainly in the short term, there is no evidence that starvation mode exists.

Indeed, when you think of it from an evolutionary perspective, "starvation mode" makes little sense. Our remote ancestors often had to go without food for longish periods, and if every time this happened they became less active and waited for pizza to be delivered, they would have become extinct. Only during periods of prolonged famine would it make sense to slow the metabolism down and wait for better times to come.

Will my blood sugar fall, leaving me feeling faint?

In the trial mentioned above, they also measured the volunteers' blood glucose levels. The researchers found that blood glucose levels did slowly fall over the three days, from 4.9 mmols/l on day one to 3.5 mmols/l by day four. These, however, are the sort of levels you might expect to see in a healthy person who had their blood taken before breakfast. They are not, in any sense, abnormally low. At the same time, the levels of fatty acids in their blood shot up, showing that their bodies had switched into major fat-burning mode.

Your body evolved to cope for periods without food.

Intermittent fasting can be tough, but there is no evidence it will cause you to faint. If in reasonable good health, your body is a remarkably efficient and functional machine, capable of—in fact, designed for—the effective regulation of blood sugar. If you are diabetic, consult your doctor before embarking on any dietary change.

Will intermittent fasting lead to muscle breakdown?

Another fear is that intermittent fasting could lead to protein deficiency and muscle breakdown. It is true that the body doesn't store protein, so after twenty-four hours without any protein in your diet your body will seek amino acids for essential things like building your immune system by cannibalizing existing muscle. But if your protein intake is adequate—and we actually recommend an increased protein percentage intake on fast days—then you are not going to get "muscle protein breakdown." In fact, the evidence from human studies points toward intermittent fasting being better than standard diets when it comes to muscle preservation.

I know I should stick to low-GI or low-GL foods on a fast day. So which foods are best?

As we've seen, foods with a low glycemic index or glycemic load will help keep your blood sugars stable, increasing your chances of a successful day with few calories. Vegetables and legumes are, needless to say, amazing, and you should rely on them on a fast day. Packed with nutrients, their bulk fills you up, they have relatively few calories, and they keep your blood sugar low. Carrots are a great snack, particularly with hummus dip, which scores an astonishing GI of 6 and 0 on the GL score. Fruit is handy too, though some fruits are more fast-friendly than others.

Check the GI count of your chosen fast-day foods online. The American Diabetes Association has an excellent guide on its website at www.diabetes.org.uk. Staple starchy foods, for instance, are worth scrutinizing with an eagle eye:

FOOD	GI	GL
Brown rice	48	20
White rice	76	36
Pasta (durum wheat)	40	20
Couscous	65	23
Potatoes, boiled	58	16
Potatoes, mashed	85	17
Potatoes, fried	75	22
Potatoes, baked	85	26

The biggest surprise among the staples is how great an effect baked or mashed potatoes have on blood sugars. On fast days, avoid these starchy basics and substitute plenty of greens. Fill your plate. Watch out for fruit, too. Some are your fast friends, but others will spike your blood sugar and are best left for the days when you are off duty.

FOOD	GI	GL
Strawberries	38	1
Apples	35	5
Oranges	42	5
Grapes	45	9
Pineapple	84	7
Banana	50	12
Raisins	64	30
Dates	100	42

Eating the whole fruit will keep you feeling full for longer. Strawberries, without sugar, are low GI/GL and also low in calories; no wonder many fasters eat a bowl for breakfast. The striking thing to note is the high sugar impact of raisins and dates. Avoid them on fast days.

> Eating the whole fruit will keep you feeling full for longer.

Beyond low-GI and protein foods, what else is on the 5:2 menu?

The following foods are tasty and low in calories, making them ideal for a fast day.

Vegetables: When it comes to vegetables, the sky's the limit: it's hard to overdo your greens. But do apply the 5:2 mantra of the double Vs—plenty of volume, plenty of variety. Aim to include different colors, textures, tastes, shapes. Steamed broccoli contains a whole world of nutrients (including vitamin K). Green beans love a little lemon and garlic. Fennel is great if shaved (invest in a mandoline), perhaps with orange segments and a squeeze of the juice. Edamame is a good source of low-fat protein and omega-3 fatty acids. Starchy veggies, of course, tend to have a higher GL and calorific value, though they are satiating. Proceed with caution and don't add butter.

Leaves: It goes without saying that green leafy veggies are your fast-day friends. Spinach, kale, chard, salad leaves . . . a veritable vitamin fest, and agreeably low in calories. Pep things up with chili flakes, ginger, cumin, pepper, lemon juice, garlic.

Fruit: Citrus fruits in general, and tangerines in particular, contain high concentrations of nobiletin, a compound that "protects from obesity and atherosclerosis"—in lab mice at least.[16] If you like tangerines, eat them, perhaps spending time meditatively peeling away the pith. The same group of researchers previously found that grapefruit, rich in a compound called naringenin, encourages the liver to burn fat rather than store it.[17] Grapefruit also contains compounds such as liminoids and lycopene (thought to have anticancer properties),[18] and clocks in at only 39 calories per half, making it a good fast-day food. (You should, however, be aware that grapefruit interacts with a number of common medicines, so if you are taking medication such as statins, consult your doctor.) Alternatively, you could always throw in a watermelon slice (30 calories per 100 grams, about 3½ ounces) or an apple (around 50 calories per 3½ ounces) for flavor, crunch, and pectin, a soluble fiber that can't be absorbed by the body but is useful in fat digestion.[19] Apples are the ultimate convenience food, though they are quite high in calories; eat the whole thing, skin, seeds, and core. Tomatoes also contain lycopene, which may help guard against cancer[20] and stroke.[21] A handful of cherry tomatoes or strawberries (low GI, low GL) could be your best bet to get you through a tummy rumble unscathed.

Berries: Blueberries are high in antioxidant polyphenols and phytonutrients. New research has found that they may also be able to break down fat cells in the body and prevent new ones from forming.[22] Even if you don't buy the science, blueberries remain a handy source of vitamin C.

Nuts: We've established that nuts are a fast-day favorite: filling and low GI. Almonds, though calorific, are high in protein and fiber, which makes them brilliantly satiating; pistachios, too (better yet, they take ages to crack and eat). Cashews and coconut flakes will help animate a salad. But count wisely; nut calories soon add up.

Cereals: Oats are a standby low-GL staple, but mix it up; you could experiment with bulgur, couscous, or quinoa—they're high in protein and fiber, easy to cook, and a good source of iron.

Dairy: Milk products, though full of protein and calcium, can also be high in fat. Perhaps opt for low-fat alternatives—and save the cheese board for tomorrow. Fat-free yogurt contains protein, potassium, and—if you want them—will bring probiotics, and, like nuts, will help you feel fuller longer. But beware; it can also be high in sugar.

Herbs and spices: Lo-cal, high-impact, no brainer. Pickles may work for you too—cornichons, jalapeños, onions (watch the GI values)—or mustard; anything, really, that brings a bolt of fire or flavor to your plate.

Soup: Scientists at Penn State University have found that soup is a great appetite suppressant.[23] Go for a light broth rather than a meaty, creamy soup to keep the calories in check.

> Whatever you eat on a fast day (or any day), the most important thing is to relish it. Go slow.

Whatever you eat on a fast day (or any day), the most important thing is to relish it. Go slow. Have a look at the menu plans on pages 145–192 for more ideas; on pages 205–210 you'll find a quick calorie counter for 150 key fast day foods.

I know I need plenty of veggies, but should I eat them raw or cooked?

There is some debate as to whether vegetables are best eaten raw or cooked; cooking may, as raw foodists contend, destroy vitamins, minerals, and enzymes, but it also softens cellulose fibers, making nutrients more available for take-up in the body. Lycopene, a potent antioxidant found in tomatoes, is boosted in cooking.[24] A small blob of ketchup is no bad thing. Meanwhile, boiled or steamed carrots, spinach, mushrooms, asparagus, cabbage, peppers, and many other vegetables supply more antioxidants, such as carotenoids and ferulic acid, to the body than they do when raw.[25] The downside of cooking vegetables is that it can destroy their vitamin C. The raw versus cooked argument is a complicated one. Our best advice? Eat plenty of vegetables, just the way you like them.

Can I eat what I like on off-duty days?

Counterintuitive as it may seem, no foods are off-limits, none forbidden. On the five days a week when we're not restricting calories, we both eat freely—fish and chips, roast potatoes, cookies, cake.

The whole point of the 5:2 approach is that for five days a week you shouldn't feel as if you are on a diet. Even so, don't try to gorge in a bid to make up for lost time, like a contestant in a blueberry pie contest. You could compensate for fasting by grossly overeating the next day, but it's very hard to do and you probably won't want to. We are creatures of habit, which makes it difficult for us to change our ways. But ingrained habits can also be helpful—after a fast people seem to find it relatively easy to step back into normal eating.

This absence of "hyperphagia" (excessive appetite) after a day of rationing calories may seem surprising, but it is borne out by anecdotal experience. Many fasters report not feeling particularly hungry the day after a fast; what's more, many people discover that their lifelong love of high-sugar, high-fat foods seems to diminish as intermittent fasting becomes a way of life. As yet, we can only speculate as to why this may be the case, but some individuals certainly experience a galvanizing effect from the weight loss they achieve: as they drop the pounds, their resolve grows stronger and they eat more healthily, and cutting back on pizzas, pies, and potatoes seems a natural lifestyle change.

Humans have, however, evolved to prefer calorie-rich foods—it once gave us an edge—and perhaps the greatest advantage of the FastDiet is that it allows pleasure foods on five days of the week. For most of the time, there is no deprivation, no guilt. The psychological impact of *not* being in denial is huge; it frustrates what's known as the "disinhibition effect"—a paradox where designating certain foods off-limits makes us likely to eat more of them.[26]

Remember, then, that this is not a cycle of bingeing and starving: it is calibrated and moderate. Studies and experience show that intermittent fasting will regulate the appetite, not make it more extreme. You could pig out on your nonfast days, working your way steadily through all the ice cream flavors in the freezer (even if you did, you'd still get some of the metabolic benefits of fasting). But you won't do that. In all likelihood, you'll remain gently, intuitively attentive to your calorie intake, almost without noticing.

Similarly, you may find yourself naturally favoring healthier foods once your palate is modified by your occasional fasts. So yes, eat freely, forbid nothing, but trust your body to say "when." In short, on a nonfast day:

★ Eat until "reasonably" full.

★ Include the occasional treat.

Is breakfast vital?

Dieting lore has long suggested that breakfast is the most important meal of the day—miss it in the morning and it's like leaving the house without a coat. But is it true?

One way to find out is to take two groups of people, breakfast skippers and breakfast eaters, and make them swap habits. Get the breakfast skippers to eat breakfast and vice versa. In a recent study, researchers did just that.[27] They recruited three hundred overweight volunteers and asked the breakfast skippers to eat breakfast, while those who routinely ate breakfast were asked to skip it. There was high compliance with the new regimens; so what actually happened?

Well, the habitual breakfast skippers who had made themselves eat breakfast lost an average of 1½ pounds. That is not a huge amount, but it is consistent with what breakfast advocates might expect. Except that the habitual breakfast eaters, who had spent 16 weeks skipping breakfast, lost an almost identical amount. The researchers concluded that, contrary to widely held belief, a recommendation to eat breakfast "had no discernible effect on weight loss in free-living adults who were attempting to lose weight."

If you are one of those people who doesn't like eating breakfast and who, perhaps, finds that eating breakfast first thing makes you hungrier, then there seems no compelling scientific reason to make yourself eat it.

What can I drink on a fast day?

Plenty—as long as it doesn't carry a substantial calorie content. In practice, as with most decisions on the FastDiet, the choice is entirely up to you. Drink lots of water—it's calorie-free, *actually* free, more filling than you think, and will stop you from confusing thirst for hunger. In summer, add rounds of cucumber or a dash of lime. Freeze it and suck on cubes. If you want warmth, miso soup contains protein, feels like food, and clocks in at only about 40 calories per cup; vegetable bouillon pulls off the same trick. A mug of instant low-cal hot chocolate, made with water? Under 40 calories and a comforting thought. No-cal drinks are better still. Hot water with lemon is a standby favorite for fasters, but you might prefer to add mint leaves or a scattering of cloves, a slice of ginger, or some lemongrass. If you are fond of herbal teas, try some unfamiliar flavors to spice up the day (licorice and cinnamon, lemongrass and ginger, lavender, rose and chamomile . . .). Try fruit teas chilled in the fridge. Green tea may have health-giving antioxidant properties (the jury's out), but if you like it, drink it.

On fast days, we drink our tea and coffee black and sugarless; if you prefer it with milk and artificial sweeteners, fine. A small glass of milk is in fact a healthier drink than, say, orange juice, being rich in protein and relatively low in carbohydrates. But beware that the calories in milk add up, and what you are trying to do is extend the time you are not consuming any calories at all.

While fruit juices are seen as healthy, they generally have a surprisingly high sugar content, are lower in fiber than a whole fruit, and can rack up the stealth calories without so much as a by-your-leave. Commercial smoothies can have a similar sugar content to Coke and, because they are acidic, they are corrosive to your teeth; they are also loaded with calories. If you need flavor, swap juice and smoothies for very dilute cordials—perhaps a dash of elderflower with fizzy water and lots of ice.

Can I have Diet Coke?

If it's the only thing that sustains you and your temper during a fast, then fine. But, counterintuitive as it may seem, studies suggest that consuming zero-calorie sweeteners such as those found in diet drinks *increases* the risk of putting on weight[28] because they provide an "orosensory stimulus," which convinces the body that a deluge of calories is about to come its way. When the advertised calories don't materialize, the system becomes confused—and as a result "people eat more or expend less energy than they otherwise would." The findings are open to debate: perhaps the best approach would be to limit intake, swapping in sparkling water instead.

What about alcohol?

Alcoholic drinks, though pleasant, merely provide empty calories. One glass of white wine contains about 120 calories, while a 12-ounce can of beer racks up 153. Unless you really can't say no, abstain absolutely on a fast day—it's a golden opportunity to slash your weekly consumption without feeling deprived. Think of it as going cold turkey for two achievable days each week.

And caffeine?

There's a growing body of evidence to suggest that far from being a guilty pleasure, drinking coffee may be good for you, helping to prevent mental decline, improve cardiac health, and reduce the risk of liver cancer and stroke.[29] So go ahead, drink coffee if that's what gets you going and keeps you going each day. It's a useful weapon in your arsenal against boredom, and a coffee break makes a happy punctuation to the day. There's no metabolic reason to avoid caffeine during a fast, but if you have trouble sleeping, limit your intake later in the day. You should, of course, drink it black. A 16-ounce caramel macchiato has 224 calories . . . just saying.

How about snacks?

The general idea of the FastDiet is to give your body an occasional holiday from eating. Let your mouth rest. Give your belly a break. All calories count on a fast day, and your objective is to achieve as long a "fasting window" as possible. Having a complete moratorium on snacking, though challenging, actually makes the process easier to handle: if "no means no," then you avoid questions or calorie calculations. No nibbles, no quibbles.

If you absolutely must snack on a fast day, do it with awareness and frugality: choose something that will not serve to elevate your insulin levels. Try a few apple slices or some strawberries. Try carrot or celery sticks with hummus, or a handful of nuts—always factor them into your daily calorie count (don't cheat); for a full list of fast-friendly snacks, see pages 188–189. And always keep an eye on the GI.

FOOD	GI	GL
Nuts	27	3
Popcorn	72	8
Rice cakes	80	19
Fruit bars	93	20
Mars bar	65	26

You knew that chocolate bars were hardly a health food, but did you know how sugary fruit bars and even some rice cakes can be? Bear in mind that processed foods tend to have hidden sugars and, though convenient, won't give you anything like the nutritional advantage of good old-fashioned plants and proteins.

Habitual snacking, even on low-calorie, nutrient-rich foods, is not advised; part of the motive here is to retrain your appetite, so don't overstimulate it. If your mouth is desperate for attention, give it a drink.

Can I use meal replacement shakes to get me through the early days?

A number of people who have tried fasting say that commercially available meal replacement shakes helped them get through the first, and normally hardest, weeks of an intermittent fast. Arguably, shakes are simpler than calorie counting, and on your fast day you simply sip away when waves of hunger strike. We are not great fans, as we think real food is better, but if you find they help, then by all means use them. It's best to go for a brand that is low in sugar.

What are the implications of cheating and having a few chips or a cookie?

To clarify: this is about fasting, the voluntary abstention from eating food. The reasons this is good for you go way beyond the fact that you are simply eating fewer calories. The benefits arise because our bodies are designed for intermittent fasts. As you've seen, what does not kill you makes you stronger. So while starvation is bad, a little bit of short, sharp, shock food restriction is good.

Your aim, then, is to carve out a food-free breathing space for your body. Going to 510 calories (or 615 for a man) won't hurt—it won't obliterate the fast. Indeed, the idea of slashing calories to a quarter of your daily intake on a fast day is simply one that has been proven to have systemic effects on the metabolism. While there's no particular magic to 500 or 600 calories, do try to stick to these numbers; you need clear parameters to make the strategy effective in the medium term.

Having a cookie on a fast day would be antithetical to your goals (not to mention the fact that it would probably spike your blood sugar and eat up most of your allowance in one buttery bite); when you're fasting, you need to think sensibly and coherently about your food choices, following the plan laid out here. Exercise willpower, reminding yourself that tomorrow is on its way.

What tests can I do to monitor changes?

Weigh yourself, of course, and measure your waist, chest, and hips once or twice a week, keeping a note of progress (you'll find a simple tracker on our website). Some weighing machines will also give you an estimate of your body fat. You could also take a measure of your resting pulse, particularly if you are combining 5:2 with exercise, as this is a good predictor of future health. You could ask your doctor to measure fasting glucose and cholesterol, and take your blood pressure.

Will I get enough nutrients in my diet?

Yes. Remember: you fast only for short periods, only occasionally. During this time, you'll eat satiating and nutritious foods, low in fat and sugar. If you stick to the tenets of the FastDiet, eating reasonably and normally on nonfast days, your diet should be nutritionally sound.

Should I take supplements during my fast?

The FastDiet is an intermittent method, not a deprivation regimen, so your nutritional intake from a wide variety of food sources should remain relatively steady over time, providing all the vitamins and minerals you require. If, as recommended, your fast-day foods center on protein and plants, they'll give you all the goodness you need without resorting to costly bottled multivitamins. Do, however, choose your fast-day foods with care, ensuring that over the course of a week you consume adequate B vitamins, omega-3s, calcium, and iron. Be sensible and eat well. While we are no fans of bottled vitamins and minerals, if a qualified health professional has suggested a particular supplement, you should continue to take it.

I've read about "superfoods" and "intelligent eating." Should I include superfoods during a fast day?

The term "superfood" is more of a marketing ploy than a scientific construct, and clinical nutritionists are loath to use the description. All plants produce a huge range of phytochemicals that can have a beneficial role in the body: eat them on a fast day or, indeed, on any day you please.

Should I exercise on a fast day?

Why not? As you will have gathered by now, we FastDieters are also keen on FastExercise (more on this in Part Two of this book). Research has shown that even a more extreme three-day total fast has no negative effect on the ability to perform short-term, high-intensity workouts or long-duration, moderate-intensity exercise. Athletes seem to suffer no loss in performance during occasional fasting; a 2008 study of Tunisian footballers during Ramadan found that fasting had no effect on performance. ("Each player was assessed for speed, power, agility, endurance, and for passing and dribbling skills. No variables were negatively affected by fasting.")[30]

In fact—and this is worth noting if you are aiming for optimal fitness—training while fasting can result in better metabolic adaptations[31] (which means enhanced performance over time), improved muscle protein synthesis,[32] and a higher anabolic response to postexercise feeding.[33]

Training on an empty stomach turns out to be beneficial on multiple levels, coaxing the body to burn a greater percentage of fat for fuel instead of relying on recently consumed carbs; if you're burning fat, don't forget, you're not storing it. As we've seen, one recent study found that working out before breakfast is beneficial for metabolic performance and weight loss.[34] A report in the *New York Times* suggested that it even "blunts the deleterious effects of overindulging"—making fasted exercise a canny way of "combating Christmas."[35] According to the study's authors, "Our current data indicate that exercise training in the fasted state is more effective than exercise in the carbohydrate-fed state." Certainly food for thought.

Do not, however, increase your fast day food allowance to "compensate" for calories burned through exercise: on a fast day, stick to 500 or 600 calories, whatever level of activity you choose. That's where the benefits lie.

Fast 500 Menu Plans for Women

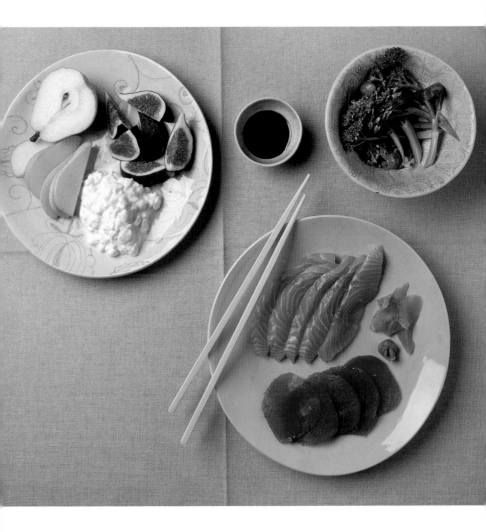

Breakfast: Cottage cheese, sliced pear, and a fresh fig.

152 calories

(See page 149.)

Dinner: Salmon and tuna sashimi with soy sauce, wasabi, pickled ginger, and broccoli.

341 calories

(See page 149.)

Total calorie count: 493

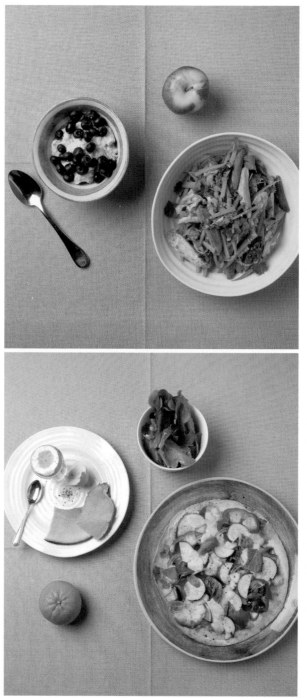

Breakfast: Oatmeal with fresh blueberries.

175 calories

(See page 150.)

Dinner: Chicken stir-fry.

360 calories

(See page 150.)

Total calorie count: 535

Breakfast: Ham and egg.

140 calories

(See page 155.)

Dinner: Tortilla pizza.

359 calories

(See page 155.)

Total calorie count: 499

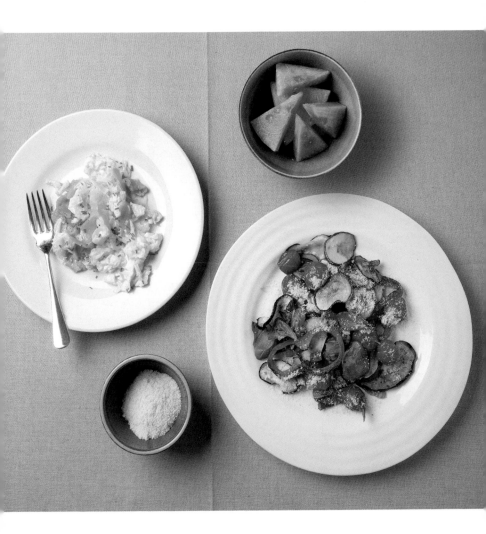

Breakfast: Scrambled eggs with smoked salmon.

216 calories

(See page 156.)

Dinner: Warm vegetable salad.

272 calories

(See page 156.)

Total calorie count: 488

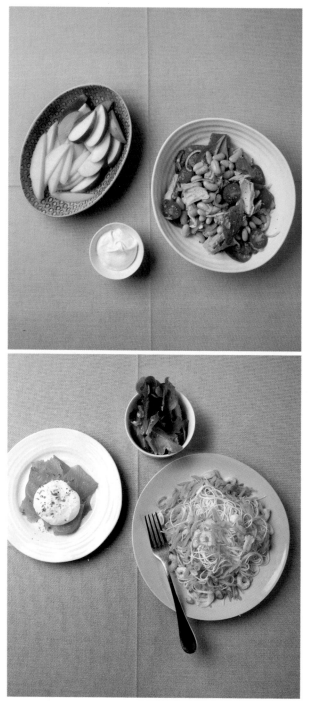

Breakfast: Apple and mango with dip.

245 calories

(See page 154.)

Dinner: Tuna and bean salad.

257 calories

(See page 154.)

Total calorie count: 502

Breakfast: Poached egg and smoked salmon.

220 calories

(See page 152.)

Dinner: Thai salad

275 calories

(See page 152.)

Total calorie count: 495

Fast 600 Menu Plans for Men

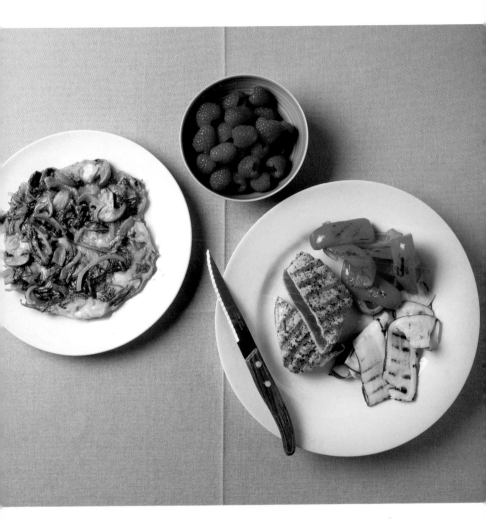

Breakfast: Mushroom and spinach frittata and a bowl of raspberries.

270 calories

(See page 159.)

Dinner: Seared tuna with grilled vegetables.

333 calories

(See page 159.)

Total calorie count: 603

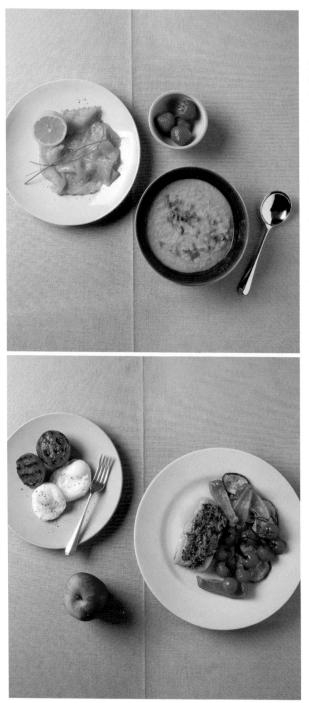

Breakfast: Smoked salmon with lemon wedges.

134 calories

(See page 168.)

Dinner: Bacon and butterbean soup.

467 calories

(See page 168.)

Total calorie count: 601

Breakfast: Poached eggs with grilled tomato.

198 calories

(See page 160.)

Dinner: Pesto salmon.

400 calories

(See page 160.)

Total calorie count: 598

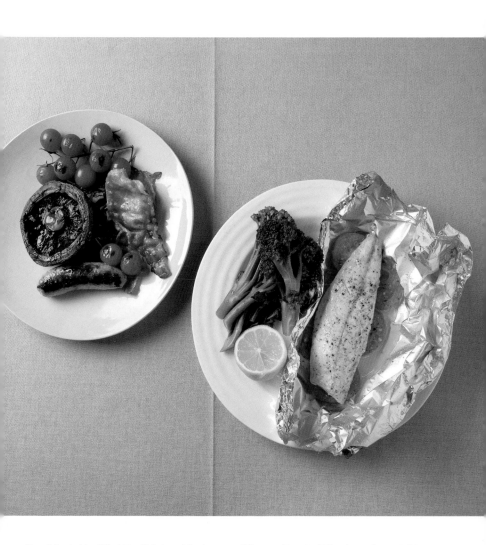

Breakfast: Modified English breakfast.

211 calories

(See page 163.)

Dinner: Roasted tilapia and vegetables.

384 calories

(See page 163.)

Total calorie count: 595

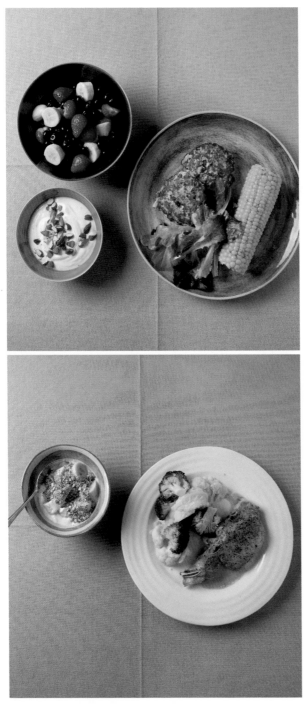

Breakfast: Yogurt with fruit and almonds.

298 calories

(See page 164.)

Dinner: Cumin-turkey burgers with corn on the cob.

324 calories

(See page 164.)

Total calorie count: 622

Breakfast: Yogurt with muesli and banana.

205 calories

(See page 167.)

Dinner: Roast pork with broccoli and cauliflower.

383 calories

(See page 167.)

Total calorie count: 588

Are there gender differences in response to intermittent fasting?

Clearly, men and women have metabolic and hormonal differences; for evolutionary reasons, we store and utilize fat in different ways. Women carry more fat, are better at storing it, and tend to be more efficient at burning fat in response to exercise.[36]

Though few studies have been done, there's some evidence to suggest that fasting women have a better response to endurance training than weight training,[37] while men may fare better with weights. Anecdotally, men tend to find working out on an empty stomach easier to accomplish than women.

In terms of general health, the benefits of occasional, short-term fasting for both sexes are pretty clear. Although quite a few human studies have been done with male volunteers, others have been done with a mixed group or mainly female volunteers. The volunteers who took part in Dr. Michelle Harvie's studies, well over two hundred of them, were all women. Their results are striking and positive, though further trials are required to analyze the precise effects of fasting on hormones, particularly among women of different ages. As with all recommendations in this book, be cautious and self-aware. Fasting is not meant to be a struggle; it's intended as a well-marked route to good health. If, for whatever reason, short bouts of fasting interrupt your menstrual cycle or your sleep pattern, modify your approach till you find a comfortable balance that works for you.

Should I fast during my period?

Some women may find fasting more challenging on the days preceding a period; we don't yet have any clear studies on the impact of intermittent fasting on the menstrual cycle, but if you feel this may be the case for you, perhaps embark in the days following the start of your period, not before.

Can I fast if I'm trying to get pregnant?

The science is still unfolding, and there haven't been enough clinical trials to assess the overall effects of fasting on fertility. According to Professor Mark Mattson, an intermittent fasting plan such as the FastDiet will not affect fertility. More extreme fasting may. It does in animals, but in a reversible manner. Nonetheless, we err on the side of caution and suggest that if you are trying to get pregnant, you should not fast.

Who else shouldn't fast?

There are certain groups for whom fasting is not advised. These are:

★ Children: they are still growing and should not be subject to nutritional stress of any kind

★ Type-1 diabetics and diabetics on insulin

★ Pregnant women and breast-feeding mothers, who should eat according to government guidelines and not limit their calorie intake

★ Anyone with an eating disorder, and the very lean or underweight

★ People recovering from surgery, and those with an underlying medical condition or taking prescribed medications (we would advise you to see your doctor first, as you would before embarking on any weight-loss regimen)

★ Anyone feeling unwell or feverish: fasting will stress your body, which seems to be one of the ways that it is effective (stress, as we've seen, provokes repair), but you shouldn't *over* stress

★ If you are taking warfarin: consult your doctor first as it may increase your INR

Will I get headaches?

If you do, it may be due to dehydration rather than a lack of calories. You might experience mild withdrawal symptoms from sugar (or caffeine, if you've dropped it), but the brevity of your fast shouldn't make this of special concern. Keep drinking water. Treat a headache as you otherwise would; if fasting today is making you feel particularly unwell, stop. You are in charge.

Will I become constipated?

If constipation is an issue, it's often the result of not drinking enough water. So stay hydrated. Try adding psyllium husk to your diet. If the problem persists, consult your GP.

Will I feel tired?

Short-term, deliberate, modified fasting should not exhaust you—some fasters even report an energy boost on a fast day and beyond. As in normal life, you'll undoubtedly have up days and down days, good days and bad. See how you fare. You may find that a fast day ends sooner than most—an early night, no alcohol, and plentiful sleep being a great way to arrive at breakfast sooner.

Will I feel cold?

Some people, my father included, do report feeling a bit cold after losing weight on the 5:2. If you have carried a fair amount of weight around for many years, almost as a comfort blanket, losing it will certainly have an effect. You could do some energetic exercise to stoke things up. Or wear an extra sweater . . .

Will I go to bed hungry?

Probably not, though it will depend on your particular metabolism, and how you timed your fast-day calorie consumption. If you feel hungry, take your mind off it—a bubble bath, a good book, a stretch out, a cup of herbal tea. Get psychology on your side: congratulate yourself on reaching the end of another fast day. Surprisingly perhaps, fasters report that they don't wake up ravenous and run for the fridge as soon as the alarm goes off. Hunger is a subtle beast, and your appetite will soon find its rhythm.

> Surprisingly perhaps, fasters report that they don't wake up ravenous and run for the fridge as soon as the alarm goes off. Hunger is a subtle beast, and your appetite will soon find its rhythm.

Will fasting affect my sleep?

Some people find it hard to sleep on a relatively empty stomach. If so, Michael recommends setting aside calories for a late-night glass of milk or small snack. There is evidence that the side effects you experience are the ones you expect, so it is best to approach intermittent fasting with the expectation that it will be fine.

Will fasting affect my gout?

Longer-term fasting can precipitate gout, but this should not occur with intermittent fasting. On the other hand, gout is associated with metabolic syndrome (obesity, insulin resistance, high cholesterol, high blood pressure) and 5:2 should help correct this, partly through weight loss but also by reducing insulin levels. In addition, as Michael has outlined above, IF seems to reduce inflammation.

What if everyone around me is eating on one of my fast days?

Participate, but with a nonchalant awareness. While support from family and friends is an asset, making a song and dance about your fast will only cause you to feel self-conscious, turning the diet into an obstruction, a hurdle, rather than something that should slot happily and calmly into your life. Remember your trump card: you'll eat normally again tomorrow. Some days, of course, are tougher than others. Naturally enough, you may find yourself feeling hungrier and less able to fast successfully when celebrating or attending events that revolve around food. If you know that you have a social event on your schedule, fast the day before or the day after. The flexibility of the plan explicitly means—in fact, it demands—that you still go to that wedding, birthday, anniversary dinner, christening, bar mitzvah, supper date, posh restaurant. Take a break for Christmas, Easter, Thanksgiving, Diwali. Yes, you may well put on a little weight, but this is a life, not a life sentence. You can always deviate, eat chips and dips and things on sticks, and then revert to more challenging fasting once the party's over.

What if I'm currently obese?

Clinical trials have concluded that intermittent fasting is a sustainable—indeed, one of the most effective—ways for obese individuals to lose weight and keep it off; the larger you are, the greater your initial weight loss is likely to be. If you are obese, it's likely that for whatever reasons, traditional restrictive diets have failed for you. The FastDiet is different because of its flexibility, its war on guilt, and its approval of occasional "pleasure foods" on nonfast days. Studies done by Dr. Michelle Harvie and Professor Tony Howell, cited above, have shown that most overweight women are able to adapt to calorie restricting two days a week and lose significant amounts of fat, even those who have had long-term weight issues. As with any underlying medical condition, we recommend that you fast under supervision.

Should I add a third day if I want to see accelerated results doing 4:3?

As Michael wrote earlier, there is good scientific evidence from trials run by Dr. Krista Varady and her team at the University of Illinois in Chicago of benefits from more rigorous intermittent fasting. They have done a number of carefully controlled studies where volunteers have tried alternate-day fasting (ADF). This form of intermittent fasting entails cutting calories every other day—a 500-calorie allowance for women, 600 for men. Most volunteers who took part in these studies lost significant amounts of weight, mainly as fat, and saw marked improvements in their biomarkers, including cholesterol.

I'm already slim enough, but would like to enjoy the health benefits of intermittent fasting. Is that possible?

If you are already at a reasonable, happy weight, you can still fast effectively, but consider adapting your consumption on nonfast days to encompass more calorie-dense foods. The main researchers we talked to in this field are all slim and they still fast. With practice, you will discover an amicable balance between fasting and feeding that keeps your weight in the prescribed range. As you reach your target weight, alter your routine to fast once a week, rather than twice a week. This is what we call the Maintenance Model, or 6:1.

While there have been no specific studies to illuminate the effects of doing this, there do seem to be benefits from intermittent fasting that go beyond weight loss. We know, for example, that repair and routine maintenance goes on in the cells when we are not eating; studies suggest that a day a week of calorie restriction will keep the weight off and allow you to retain significant biochemical benefits.

So, use your common sense and watch the scales; don't slide. As mentioned above, if you are already extremely lean or suffering from an eating disorder, fasting of any description is not advised. If in doubt, see your GP.

Is it too late to start?

On the contrary, there's no time to lose. The FastDiet is likely to prolong your life. It will moderate your appetite and help you lose weight. Its effects are quickly felt, often within a week of starting your simple biweekly mini-fasts. It all

The FastDiet is likely to prolong your life. It will moderate your appetite and help you lose weight. Its effects are quickly felt, often within a week of starting your simple biweekly mini-fasts.

points to a healthier, leaner, longer old age, fewer doctors' appointments, more energy, greater resistance to disease. Our advice? Start yesterday.

How long should I continue?

Interestingly, the FastDiet's on/off eating scheme looks a lot like the approach of many naturally slim people. Some days they'll pick, other days, they'll tuck into treats. In the long run, this is how the FastDiet goes. As you settle into the routine, you'll naturally moderate your calorie intake on fast days and feed days, until the process is innate. When you reach your target weight, you can change the frequency of your fast. Play with it. But don't drift; stay alert. Your aim is a permanent life change, not a blip, not a fad, not a dinner-party chat. This is a long-distance route to sustained weight loss. Accept that it is something you will do, in a form that suits you, indefinitely. For as long as life.

The future of fasting: where next?

Fasting, as we mentioned at the beginning of the book, has been practiced for many thousands of years and yet science is only just starting to catch up. The first evidence of the long-term benefits of calorie restriction were found just over eighty years ago, when nutritionists working with rats at Cornell University discovered that if you severely restrict the amount they eat, they live longer. Much longer.

Since then, the evidence has continued to mount that animals not only live longer, healthier lives if they are calorie-restricted, they also do so if they are intermittently starved. In recent years the research has moved on from rodents to humans, and we are seeing the same patterns of improvement.

So where do we go from here? Professor Valter Longo, who has done so much pioneering work with IGF-1, is running a number of human trials in conjunction with colleagues at the University of Southern California, looking at the impact of fasting on cancer. They have already demonstrated that fasting will cut your risk of developing cancer; now they want to see if fasting will also improve the efficacy of chemotherapy and radiation.

Valter Longo believes that we should try to tackle the problems of aging as a whole, rather than one disease at a time. Instead of focusing so much research money on heart disease or cancer, we should try to slow down the cellular damage that leads to the diseases of old age. Fasting, whether short term or intermittent, is clearly one way to do this.

Dr. Michelle Harvie and Professor Tony Howell, who work at the Genesis Breast Cancer Prevention Centre in Manchester, in England, have done a great deal of fascinating work developing and testing different forms of two-day intermittent energy restriction. In this book we have quoted a couple of their studies—involving hundreds of female volunteers—that have shown that people can lose weight just as effectively by calorie restricting on an intermittent basis as by calorie restricting every day. They are planning further studies, comparing what they call the "2-Day Diet" with standard dieting. These studies will undoubtedly add to our understanding of how well people are able to tolerate different patterns of eating in the long run.

Professor Mark Mattson of the National Institute on Aging in Baltimore is adding all the time to the dozens of research papers he has already published on the effects of fasting and intermittent fasting on the brain. We are particularly interested to see the outcome of some of his current studies, which include looking further into what happens to the brains of volunteers when put on an intermittent fasting regimen.

He is keen to emphasize the importance of regular exercise alongside intermittent fasting, as many of the changes you see, whether it's improving glucose regulation or the effects on the brain, are similar with exercise and intermittent fasting. Any form of exercise is better than nothing, but there is currently a lot of excitement around HIT, which seems to produce greater changes in less time.

Despite the benefits, many people may not want to fast, so there is considerable interest in developing drugs that mimic some of the effects of intermittent fasting. There is a drug called Byetta, used for the treatment of diabetes, which also activates the production of BDNF (brain-derived neurotrophic factor). This in turn, as we've seen, seems to protect the brain against the ravages of aging. The hope is that Byetta or a related drug will, if not prevent dementia, at least significantly slow its progression.

Another interesting candidate is the drug rapamycin, first isolated from bacteria found in the soil of Easter Island. Rapamycin, like fasting, acts on something called the mTor pathway, which regulates protein synthesis and cell growth. It is implicated in a range of common diseases, including diabetes, obesity, depression, and some cancers. Pharmaceutical companies are currently creating and testing modified versions of rapamycin.

Intermittent fasting has, until now, been one of the best-kept secrets in science. We look forward, with a great deal of personal interest, to seeing how this particular story unfolds.

CHAPTER THREE

Menu Plans

Fast Day Cooking Tips

1. Feel free to bump up the low-calorie, low-GI leafy vegetables beyond the quantities. It is difficult to overdo it on leafy veggies, and if you need bulk, here's where you should get it. Lightly steaming vegetables is the best cooking method. So invest in a tiered bamboo steamer, and cook your proteins and veggies in several health-packed, eco-friendly levels. Scrub vegetables rather than peel them, as many nutrients are found close to the skin. Eating the skins will add fiber to your diet. When browning and caramelizing vegetables, put them in a hot, dry pan and then spray with oil, rather than adding the oil first—this will reduce the amount of oil absorbed during cooking.

2. Some vegetables benefit from cooking; others are better eaten raw (see pages 118–119 for more details). Cooking certain vegetables—including carrots, spinach, mushrooms, asparagus, cabbage, and peppers—breaks down the cell structure without destroying vitamins, allowing you to absorb more goodies. For raw vegetables, a mandoline makes preparation easy and swift.

3. Fast days should be low-fat rather than no-fat. A teaspoon of olive oil can be used in cooking, or drizzled over vegetables for flavor, or use an olive oil spray to get a thin film. Alternatively, use a silicon brush to apply oil to the pan and dab away excess with kitchen paper. Nuts and fattier meats such as pork are included in the plans. Do include a light oil dressing on your salads; it means that you are more likely to absorb their fat-soluble vitamins.

4. The acid in lemon or orange dressings means that you will absorb more iron from leafy greens such as spinach and kale. Watercress with orange is a great combination, perhaps scattered with some sesame and sunflower seeds or blanched almonds for a little protein and crunch.

5. Eating protein will help keep you fuller longer. Stick to the low-fat proteins, including some nuts and legumes. Cooking meat and poultry with its skin on

will maximize flavor and prevent drying out, but don't eat the skin. Much of the fat lies there. Roast on a rack over a baking pan to allow excess fat to drip away. Similarly, a grill pan channels fat into the grooves and away from your plate.

6. Swap ground beef for mushrooms to lessen your calorie load, and consider extending your meat eating to include lean game. Venison, for example, has a fraction of the fat found in beef. Eggs, meanwhile, are a fast day standby; boiling or poaching them means you're not adding further calories.

7. Dairy is also included here: choose lower-fat cheeses and 1% or 2% milk; avoid full-fat yogurt in favor of low-fat alternatives. Drop the lattes and toss out the butter on a fast day—they are calorie traps.

8. Avoid starchy white carbohydrates (bread, potatoes, pasta) and opt instead for low-GI carbs such as vegetables, beans and lentils, and slow-burn whole-grain cereals. Choose brown rice and quinoa. Oatmeal for breakfast will keep you fuller for longer than cold cereal.

9. Ensure that you get some fiber in your fast: eat the skin of apples and pears, have oats for breakfast, keep those leafy vegetables coming in.

10. Add flavor where you can: red pepper flakes will give a kick to any savory dish. Vinegars, including balsamic, and lemon juice will lend acidity. Add fresh herbs, too—they are virtually calorie free but give personality to a plate.

11. Soup can be a savior on a fast day, particularly if you choose a light broth packed with leafy vegetables (miso soup would be ideal). Soup is satiating, and a good way of using up ingredients languishing in the fridge. When making a soup base, don't sweat vegetables in butter; use water or a spray of oil. Thicken with pulses instead of potatoes (a handful of lentils will do the trick), or gravitate toward clear vegetable broths; vegetable stock generally has a lower fat content than chicken stock. If it suits the recipe, leave vegetables whole rather than blitzing. Add miso, bouillon cubes, or bouillon powder to capitalize on taste.

12. Use agave as a sweetener if required; it's relatively low-GI. Or try stevia.

13. Always cook with a nonstick pan to cut down on calorie-dense fats. Add a splash of water if the food sticks.

14. Weigh your food after preparing it, so that the calorie count is correct.

Fast 500 Menu Plans for Women

Day 1

Breakfast (152 calories)
Scant ½ cup low-fat cottage cheese (78 calories)
½ sliced pear (50 calories)
1 fresh fig (24 calories)

Dinner (341 calories)

SALMON WITH TUNA SASHIMI
3 to 5 pieces each of salmon (3.5 ounces/185 calories)
and tuna sashimi (3.5 ounces/120 calories)
2 teaspoons soy sauce (2 calories)
Wasabi
Pickled ginger (9 calories)
Broccolini topped with ½ teaspoon olive oil (20
calories), a squeeze of lemon, and slices of fresh red
chile (1.7 ounces/5 calories)

Daily Total: 493 calories

Day 2

Breakfast (175 calories)

Oatmeal made with 1.4 ounces steel-cut oats (155 calories) and water

¼ cup fresh blueberries (20 calories)

Dinner (360 calories)

CHICKEN STIR-FRY

Cut a 5-ounce chicken breast fillet (175 calories) into strips. Stir-fry in a nonstick skillet in 1 teaspoon olive oil (40 calories) with 1 teaspoon finely chopped ginger (2 calories), 1 tablespoon chopped cilantro (3 calories), 1 clove garlic, crushed (3 calories), 2 teaspoons soy sauce (3 calories), and the juice of ½ small lemon (1 calorie) until the chicken is lightly browned. Add water if it sticks.

Add ½ cup trimmed snow peas (12 calories), 1½ cups shredded cabbage (26 calories), and 2 small carrots, peeled and cut into thin strips (45 calories). Stir-fry for 5 to 10 minutes more, until the chicken is cooked through. Add water if necessary. Season and serve.

1 small apple (50 calories)

Daily Total: 535 calories

Day 3

Breakfast (130 calories)

1 large boiled egg (90 calories)

½ small grapefruit (40 calories)

Dinner (383 calories)

VEGETARIAN CHILI

Fry 1 clove garlic, chopped (3 calories), and ½ large fresh red chile, seeded and finely chopped, in 1 teaspoon olive oil (40 calories) in a nonstick skillet. Add a pinch of ground cumin and 4 small white mushrooms or 1 large white mushroom, chopped (3 calories). Cook for 5 minutes, adding water if it sticks.

Stir in ½ of a 14-ounce can chopped tomatoes with juices (44 calories) and scant ½ of a 14-ounce can kidney beans, rinsed and drained (180 calories). Season and simmer for 10 minutes.

Serve with ½ cup cooked brown rice (113 calories).

Daily Total: 513 calories

Day 4

Breakfast (220 calories)
> 4 ounces smoked salmon (140 calories)
> 1 medium poached egg (80 calories)

Dinner (275 calories)

THAI SALAD

Soak 1.8 ounces rice vermicelli noodles (100 calories) in water according to package instructions.

Combine 2 tablespoons Thai fish sauce (10 calories), the juice of 1 lime (2 calories), 1 teaspoon sugar (9 calories), 2 scallions (white and green parts), trimmed and thinly sliced (5 calories), and 1 very small red chile, finely chopped (1 calorie) in a bowl. Mix well. Add 10 very small cooked and peeled shrimp (58 calories) and 3 medium carrots, peeled and grated (70 calories). Drain the noodles and add. Season, toss well, and serve with a handful of leaf salad (10 calories) dressed with a spray of olive oil and squeeze of lemon juice (10 calories).

Daily Total: 495 calories

Day 5

Breakfast (177 calories)

STRAWBERRY SMOOTHIE

Blend 1 small banana (85 calories), a ½ cup fat-free plain yogurt (62 calories), 8 strawberries (1¼-inch diameter), trimmed and hulled (30 calories), a splash of water, and some cracked ice until thick and creamy. Serve immediately.

Dinner (325 calories)

OVEN-BAKED TILAPIA

Preheat the oven or a toaster oven to 400°F. Very lightly coat a small baking dish with cooking spray. Place a 7- to 8-ounce tilapia fillet (202 calories) in the dish and sprinkle with your favorite dried herbs or ground spices. Bake for 15 to 20 minutes, until cooked through.

Serve with a large poached egg (90 calories) and ⅔ cup lightly steamed broccoli florets or chopped broccoli rabe (33 calories).

Daily Total: 502 calories

Day 6

Breakfast (245 calories)

1 small apple, sliced (50 calories)
1 small mango, peeled and pitted (95 calories)
Serve with 2 tablespoons low-fat crème fraîche dip
(100 calories)

Dinner (257 calories)

TUNA AND BEAN SALAD

Combine ½ cup canned cannellini beans, drained and
rinsed (110 calories), one 5-ounce can solid white tuna
in spring water, drained (119 calories), 2 ounces grape
tomatoes (16 calories), and 1 loosely packed cup baby
spinach (8 calories) in a salad bowl.

In a small bowl, combine 1 clove garlic, crushed
(3 calories), the juice and grated zest of lemon (1 calorie), salt and pepper, and a splash of white wine vinegar.
Drizzle over the salad and toss to mix well.

Daily Total: 502 calories

Day 7

Breakfast (140 calories)

1 medium boiled egg (80 calories)

1 small slice of 97% fat-free ham (30 calories)

1 small tangerine (30 calories)

Dinner (359 calories)

TORTILLA PIZZA

Preheat the oven or a toaster oven to 400°F. Top one 8-inch whole-wheat tortilla (144 calories) with 1 tablespoon tomato puree (5 calories) and 2 ounces fresh mozzarella cheese, diced (140 calories). Scatter with about 6 ounces chopped lightly steamed vegetables (50 calories); mushrooms, red pepper, zucchini, red onion, eggplant, spinach are all okay. Season and cook for 5 to 10 minutes. Serve topped with fresh basil leaves and a side salad of leaves drizzled with a spray of olive oil (20 calories).

Daily Total: 499 calories

Day 8

Breakfast (216 calories)

SCRAMBLED EGGS WITH SMOKED SALMON

Whisk together 2 medium eggs (160 calories) and 1 tablespoon skim milk (5 calories). Season and scramble in a dry nonstick skillet until cooked but not completely dry. Remove from the heat and stir in 1.5 ounces smoked salmon, cut in slivers (51 calories).

Dinner (272 calories)

WARM VEGETABLE SALAD

Preheat the oven or a toaster oven to 400°F. Very lightly coat a baking dish with cooking spray. In the baking dish, combine 10 cherry tomatoes (25 calories), ½ small zucchini, trimmed and sliced (15 calories), ½ cup cubed eggplant (25 calories), and 1 scant cup sliced red bell pepper (51 calories). Scatter with fresh basil leaves (1 calorie) and drizzle with ½ teaspoon balsamic vinegar (5 calories). Bake for 20 to 25 minutes, stirring occasionally, until the vegetables are softened and lightly browned. Season and serve with ¼ cup grated Parmesan cheese (80 calories).

7 ounces watermelon (70 calories)

Daily Total: 488 calories

Day 9

Breakfast (137 calories)

½ cup low-fat plain yogurt (77 calories)

¼ cup fresh blueberries (20 calories)

1 slice of 97% fat-free ham (40 calories)

Dinner (358 calories)

CHICKPEA CURRY

Heat a pan and spray with oil (10 calories). Sauté 1 small onion, chopped (27 calories), and 1 clove garlic, crushed (3 calories), for 2 minutes until softened. Add 1 teaspoon curry powder and a pinch of red pepper flakes (or to taste) and cook for another 2 minutes. Add ½ cup boiling water, 1 vegetable bouillon cube (10 calories), 1 tablespoon tomato paste (14 calories), and ½ cup canned chickpeas (132 calories). Simmer for 5 to 10 minutes. Add 5 cherry tomatoes (14 calories) and a handful of spinach leaves (8 calories) toward the end of the cooking time. Season and serve with ¾ cup brown rice (140 calories).

Daily Total: 495 calories

Day 10

Breakfast (275 calories)

SHAKSHOUKA

Heat a medium sauté pan and warm 1 teaspoon of olive oil (40 calories). Add 1 clove garlic, minced (3 calories), and cook for 5 to 7 minutes over medium heat until softened. Stir in 14.5 ounces of diced tomatoes (74 calories) and 1 tablespoon of tomato paste (14 calories), with the paprika, mild chili powder, ground cumin, a pinch of cayenne pepper, and simmer for 5 to 7 minutes more, until it starts to reduce. Season with salt and pepper, then crack 2 small eggs (140 calories) directly over the tomato mixture. Cover and cook for 10 minutes, until the egg whites are firm, the yolks are still runny, and the sauce has slightly reduced. Garnish with chopped parsley (4 calories).

Dinner (208 calories)

FAST DAY INSALATA CAPRESE

Slice 2 ounces fresh mozzarella cheese (140 calories). Slice 1 large beefsteak tomato (33 calories). Alternate the slices on a plate. Scatter with fresh basil leaves and drizzle with ½ teaspoon balsamic vinegar (5 calories).

8 large strawberries (30 calories)

Daily Total: 483 calories

600-Calories-a-Day Menus for Men

Day 1

Breakfast (270 calories)

MUSHROOM AND SPINACH FRITTATA

Sauté 1 small onion, sliced (27 calories), in 1 teaspoon olive oil (40 calories) in a nonstick skillet until translucent. Add 2 small white mushrooms or 1 large white mushroom, chopped (3 calories), and cook until the mushrooms are barely tender. Add 1 loosely packed cup baby spinach (8 calories) and cook for 2 minutes more. Pour in 2 medium eggs, beaten (160 calories). Cook undisturbed for 5 minutes, and finish under a hot broiler until the eggs are set.

2 ounces raspberries (32 calories)

Dinner (333 calories)

SEARED TUNA WITH GRILLED VEGETABLES

Cut 1 small red bell pepper, stemmed and seeded (50 calories), and 1 small zucchini, trimmed (18 calories), into slices about ¼-inch wide. Toss in a bowl with 1 teaspoon olive oil (40 calories). Season lightly. Heat a grill pan over medium-high heat and grill the vegetables 5 minutes per side, flipping the slices once. Serve on a plate and dress with a squeeze of lemon.

In the same pan, grill a 5-ounce tuna steak (225 calories), flipping once, until done to your taste. Plate with the vegetables, with another squeeze of lemon.

Daily Total: 603 calories

Day 2

Breakfast (198 calories)
  2 large poached eggs (180 calories)
  1 small grilled tomato (18 calories)

Dinner (400 calories)

PESTO SALMON

Preheat the oven to 350°F. Spread 2 teaspoons pesto (52 calories) over a 5-ounce salmon fillet (275 calories). Season and bake until the salmon is cooked through, about 15 minutes. Serve with baked veggies—½ medium zucchini, cut into ribbons (18 calories), 10 cherry tomatoes on the vine (27 calories), and ½ medium red bell pepper, cut into strips (26 calories); spray with a little oil (2 calories) and place in the oven for 6 to 8 minutes, turning halfway through.

Daily Total: 598 calories

Day 3

Breakfast (307 calories)

SPICED PEAR OATMEAL

Simmer ⅓ cup jumbo oats (104 calories), 1 cup skim milk (105 calories), and ½ medium pear, peeled and diced (47 calories), with ½ teaspoon cinnamon, and a grating of nutmeg. Stir and cook until oatmeal is thickened to your liking. Serve with 2 teaspoons chopped hazelnuts (37 calories), adding 1 teaspoon of agave nectar (14 calories) to taste.

Dinner (295 calories)

NO-CARB CAESAR SALAD

Heat a grill pan over medium-high heat. Grill 2 slices Canadian bacon (76 calories) for 4 to 5 minutes, flipping once. Set aside to cool, then coarsely chop.

Cut a 5-ounce chicken breast fillet (148 calories) in half to make two thinner fillets. Grill for 3 to 4 minutes on each side, until cooked through. Cut into cubes. Place the chicken on a bed of about 2 cups chopped romaine lettuce (16 calories). Sprinkle with 1 tablespoon grated Parmesan cheese (45 calories) and drizzle with 1 tablespoon fat-free Caesar salad dressing (10 calories). Sprinkle the bacon over the top.

Daily Total: 602 calories

Day 4

Breakfast (300 calories)

CHEESE AND TOMATO OMELET

Whisk together 2 medium eggs (160 calories) and 1 tablespoon skim milk (5 calories). Cook undisturbed in a dry nonstick skillet until set but still slightly moist on top. Top with 2 very thin slices fresh tomato (5 calories) and 1 slice American cheese (100 calories). Remove from the heat, cover, and let sit until the cheese has melted.

1 small tangerine (30 calories)

Dinner (295 calories)

MARINATED STEAK AND ASIAN COLE SLAW

Marinate a 3-ounce piece sirloin steak (145 calories) in a mixture of 1 teaspoon soy sauce (1 calorie), juice of 1 lime (2 calories), and 1 clove garlic, crushed (3 calories), for about 10 minutes. Heat a grill pan over medium-high heat. Remove steak from marinade and grill to desired doneness, turning once. Set aside to cool.

For the Asian cabbage salad: in a bowl, combine 1 small carrot, peeled and grated (28 calories), 1½ cups shredded savoy cabbage (24 calories), and a handful of cilantro sprigs, chopped (2 calories). In a separate bowl, combine 1 teaspoon sugar (16 calories) with 1 tablespoon Thai fish sauce (10 calories), juice of 1 lime (1 calorie), and 1 clove garlic, crushed (3 calories). Pour over the salad and toss to combine. Arrange on plate. Slice steak and arrange on salad. Top with 1 tablespoon chopped unsalted dry-roasted peanuts (60 calories).

Daily Total: 595 calories

Day 5

Breakfast (211 calories)

MODIFIED ENGLISH BREAKFAST
Cook 1½ strips thick-sliced bacon (107 calories) until crisp. Heat 1 small brown 'n' serve sausage (59 calories). Grill 10 cherry tomatoes (27 calories) and 1 small portobello mushroom cap (10 calories). Arrange on top of 1 loosely packed cup baby spinach (8 calories), sautéed for 2 minutes in a pan with a dash of boiling water. Dry spinach thoroughly and season well with salt and pepper.

Dinner (384 calories)

ROASTED TILAPIA AND VEGETABLES
Preheat the oven or a toaster oven to 400°F. Lay out a square of foil and very lightly coat it with cooking oil spray. Arrange 2 medium tomatoes, sliced (30 calories), on the foil and top with a 6-ounce tilapia fillet (320 calories). Bring two opposite corners of the foil together and

fold over tightly. Repeat with the other corners to make a tight packet. Roast for 10 to 15 minutes, or until fish is cooked through. Place the packet on a plate and open carefully.

Serve with ⅔ cup lightly steamed broccoli florets or chopped broccoli rabe (33 calories), dressed with juice of ½ lemon (1 calorie) and a light sprinkle of salt.

Daily Total: 595 calories

Day 6

Breakfast (298 calories)
½ cup low-fat plain yogurt (77 calories)
1 small banana, sliced (85 calories)
4 medium strawberries (16 calories)
½ cup blueberries (40 calories)
6 almonds, chopped (80 calories)

Dinner (324 calories)

CUMIN-TURKEY BURGERS WITH CORN ON THE COB
Combine 4 ounces ground dark turkey (123 calories), 1 medium scallion, finely chopped (2 calories), 1 tablespoon of egg, beaten (35 calories), ½ small red chile, finely chopped (9 calories), 1 clove garlic, minced (3 calories), ½ teaspoon ground cumin, ½ teaspoon ground coriander, salt, and pepper. Let marinate for ½ hour in

the fridge. Shape into 2 patties and grill for 5 to 7 minutes on each side, until cooked through. Serve with 2 cups lemon-dressed salad leaves (20 calories) and corn on the cob, boiled and dusted with paprika (132 calories).

Daily total: 622 calories

Day 7

Breakfast (261 calories)

SCRAMBLED EGGS
Whisk together 2 large eggs (180 calories) and 1 tablespoon skim milk (5 calories). Scramble in a dry nonstick skillet until cooked to your desired doneness. Serve with 2.5 ounces 97% fat-free sliced ham (76 calories).

Dinner (329 calories)

SPICED DAL WITH NAAN
Sauté ½ small onion, thinly sliced (14 calories), 1 clove garlic, crushed (3 calories), and 1 teaspoon finely chopped ginger (3 calories) in 1 teaspoon olive oil (40 calories) in a small saucepan for 5 minutes, until the onion is translucent. Add 1 cup water, ¼ cup red lentils, picked over and rinsed (159 calories), and a pinch each of ground cumin, ground coriander, ground turmeric, cayenne pepper, salt, and pepper. Bring to a boil, lower the heat

to medium-low, and simmer for 20 minutes, or until the lentils are tender.

Garnish with ⅓ cup fat-free plain yogurt (40 calories) and a handful of cilantro. Serve with half a low-fat naan bread (70 calories).

Daily Total: 590 calories

Day 8

Breakfast (253 calories)
2 large soft-boiled eggs (180 calories)
5 lightly steamed asparagus spears (33 calories), to dip
2 small plums (40 calories)

Dinner (359 calories)

THAI STEAK SALAD
Grill a 5-ounce sirloin steak (188 calories) until cooked to your preferred doneness. Set aside to cool to room temperature. Slice the steak very thin across the grain.

In a bowl, combine 2 cups shredded romaine lettuce (14 calories) and 1 cup shredded savoy cabbage (24 calories), a handful of bean sprouts (17 calories), and 2 small shredded carrots (45 calories). In a separate bowl, combine the juice of 1 lime (1 calorie), 1 teaspoon sugar (16 calories), 1 clove garlic, crushed (3 calories), 1 very small red chile, seeded and finely chopped (1 calorie),

1 teaspoon sesame oil (40 calories), and 1 tablespoon Thai fish sauce (10 calories). Pour over the salad and toss to combine. Place the salad on a plate and arrange the steak slices on top.

Daily Total: 612 calories

Day 9

Breakfast (205 calories)
   ½ cup fat-free plain yogurt (62 calories)
   1 medium banana, sliced (95 calories)
   1 tablespoon sugar-free muesli, not granola, stirred
      through (48 calories)

Dinner (383 calories)

ROAST PORK
   4.5 ounces sliced lean roast pork loin (289 calories)
   1 tablespoon defatted pan juices (60 calories)
   ½ cup steamed cauliflower florets (17 calories)
   ⅓ cup steamed chopped broccoli (17 calories)

Daily Total: 588 calories

Day 10

Breakfast (134 calories)

4 ounces smoked salmon (132 calories)
Lemon wedges and chopped chives to serve (2 calories)

Dinner (467 calories)

BACON AND BUTTERBEAN SOUP

Fry 2 strips bacon, chopped (116 calories) in 1 teaspoon olive oil (40 calories) in a saucepan for 2 minutes, until the fat starts to render out. Add ½ small onion, finely chopped (14 calories), 3 tablespoons chopped leek (11 calories), ½ carrot, peeled and thinly sliced (14 calories), and 1 medium stalk celery, chopped (6 calories). Cook for 5 minutes, until the onions are translucent, adding a splash of water if it sticks. Add 1 cup canned butterbeans or lima beans, drained and rinsed (240 calories), 1 cup water, and ½ of a vegetable bouillon cube (10 calories). Bring to a boil, then lower the heat and simmer for 20 minutes, until the beans are very soft. Season to taste.

Transfer the mixture to a blender and puree until the desired consistency, or mash with a potato masher for a chunkier texture.

4 medium strawberries (16 calories)

Daily Total: 601 calories

The FastDiet's Greatest Hits

Over the past few years, some recipes from *The FastDiet* cookbooks have emerged as firm favorites—chiefly because they are quick, easy, tasty, and surprisingly low in calories, while staying packed full of flavor. Here, then, are our top ten dishes to include in your 5:2 repertoire; note that some are best cooked for two or for four people, so the calories listed here are *per portion*.

Spiced Chicken with Warm Lentils and Roasted Garlic

399 calories per portion

Serves 4

FOR THE MARINADE

1½-inch-piece ginger, grated

1 teaspoon ground coriander

1 teaspoon ground cumin

1 teaspoon paprika

1 teaspoon ground turmeric

Juice of 1 lemon

2 teaspoons olive oil

Salt and pepper

1 medium chicken (about 3 pounds)

1 head garlic, sliced crosswise

4 ounces French green lentils, washed

2 tablespoons water
Generous handful parsley, chopped
Generous handful cilantro leaves, chopped
1 tablespoon snipped chives
Juice of ½ lemon
Salt and pepper

Whisk the marinade ingredients and rub into the chicken, working under the skin. Refrigerate for 1 hour, or overnight if possible. Preheat the oven to 350°F. Place the chicken and garlic in a roasting pan and roast for 1 hour 10 minutes, or until the juices run clear. Remove the chicken and garlic from the oven and rest on a separate plate, retaining the juices in the pan. While the chicken is cooking, place the lentils in a saucepan, cover with water, and boil; when cooked but still al dente, drain and rinse with cold water, drain again, and add them to the roasting pan along with 2 tablespoons water. Heat through, scraping the pan for sticky bits on the base. Remove from the heat and add the herbs and lemon juice. Stir well, season, and serve with the torn chicken (skin removed) and soft garlic.

Goan Eggplant Curry
173 calories per portion (250 calories with basmati rice)

Serves 2

1 teaspoon cumin seeds, toasted and ground
2 teaspoons coriander seeds, toasted and ground

½ teaspoon cayenne pepper
½ teaspoon ground turmeric
1 green bell pepper, seeded and finely sliced
2 cloves garlic, crushed
1¼-inch-piece ginger, grated
¾ cup water
1¼ cups low-fat coconut milk
1 tablespoon tamarind paste
1 large eggplant, cut lengthwise into 2-inch-thick slices
Salt and pepper

Place the cumin and coriander seeds in a large saucepan along with the cayenne, turmeric, bell pepper, garlic, ginger, and the water. Bring to a simmer, then add the coconut milk and tamarind paste. Cook on low heat for 10 minutes, stirring occasionally, until slightly thickened. Heat the broiler to medium-high. Place the eggplant on a foil-lined baking tray and brush with a little of the curried sauce. Broil until they are soft and cooked through, turning once and brushing the other side with the sauce, 10 to 15 minutes in total. Arrange the eggplant in a serving dish, and spoon on the rest of the hot curry sauce. Season to taste. Serve with ½ cup brown basmati rice per person.

Vietnamese Shrimp Pho
48 calories per portion (add 10 to 15 calories for every ⅓ cup of additional vegetables)

Serves 4

>   2 lemongrass stalks, outer leaves removed, inner stem
>   finely chopped
>   2 teaspoons grated fresh ginger
>   4 Kaffir lime leaves, torn
>   6 cups vegetable or fish stock
>   1 teaspoon palm sugar or light brown sugar
>   3 tablespoons Thai fish sauce
>   Juice of 1 lime
>   10 large shrimp, shelled and deveined
>   1.5 ounces bean sprouts
>   Fresh Thai basil leaves, mint, cilantro, red chili pepper
>   to serve

Use a mortar and pestle to grind the lemongrass, ginger, and lime leaves. Put the paste in a large saucepan with the stock and boil for 10 minutes. Add the sugar, fish sauce, and lime juice, tasting to check for balance. Cook the shrimp in the broth until they are pink, 2 to 3 minutes. Add the bean sprouts, plenty of herbs, and a red chile to serve.

Skinny Spaghetti Bolognese
180 calories per portion

Serves 4

Cooking spray
14 ounces lean ground beef
1 large onion, diced
1 clove garlic, crushed
1 medium celery stalk, diced
1 medium red bell pepper, diced
7 ounces mushrooms, chopped
½ teaspoon dried mixed herbs
1 teaspoon mixed spice (cumin, coriander, nutmeg)
1 (14-ounce) can diced tomatoes
3 tablespoons tomato paste
1 medium zucchini, diced
Scant 1 cup beef stock or boiling water plus bouillon
    cube
Salt and pepper

Spray a large pan with a little oil, then sauté the meat until browned and set aside in a bowl. Add the onion, garlic, celery, and bell pepper to the pan and cook gently for 2 to 3 minutes, until softened. Add the mushrooms, herbs, mixed spice, tomatoes, and tomato paste and cook for another 3 minutes. Add the browned meat and zucchini together with the stock. Cover and simmer, stirring occasionally, for 30 minutes—longer if possible to enrich the sauce. Check the seasoning and serve.

Instead of pasta, serve with . . .

★ steamed broccoli and cauliflower florets
(+35 calories per 3.5 ounces)

★ veggie "noodles"—stir-fried ribbons of zucchini,
carrot, and leek (+35 calories per 3.5 ounces)

Super-Fast Thai Green Chicken Curry
331 calories per portion

Serves 2

1¾ cups low-fat coconut milk
1 tablespoon Thai green curry paste
Scant ½ cup chicken stock
1 tablespoon lime juice
1 tablespoon Thai fish sauce
7 ounces chicken breast, cut into strips
7 ounces vegetables (choose from baby "pea" eggplant,
baby zucchini, baby corn, snow peas, broccoli
florets, bok choy, thinly sliced peppers, green beans,
shiitake or oyster mushrooms, bean sprouts, frozen
baby peas, or spinach)
1 green chile, finely sliced
Handful of fresh cilantro leaves
Lime wedges to serve

Heat 1 tablespoon of the coconut milk in a pan, stir in the
curry paste, and cook for 2 minutes to release the flavor
of the paste. Add the remaining coconut milk, the stock,
lime juice, and fish sauce. Bring to a simmer and cook

for 10 minutes. Add the chicken strips and vegetables of your choice, and continue to simmer until chicken is cooked through, about 5 minutes. Top with fresh chile and cilantro, and serve with a wedge of lime.

Huevos Rancheros

283 calories per portion

Serves 1

> 1 teaspoon olive oil
> 2 scallions, finely chopped
> 1 medium red bell pepper, sliced
> ¼ teaspoon red pepper flakes
> ¾ cup canned diced tomatoes
> 1 teaspoon balsamic vinegar
> 2 large eggs
> Handful flat-leaf parsley, coarsely chopped
> Salt and pepper

Heat oil in a small frying pan and sauté the scallions, bell pepper, and red pepper flakes for 3 minutes. Add the tomatoes and vinegar. Season, stir, and simmer for 5 minutes. Make two dips in the sauce and crack an egg into each. Continue cooking until the whites have begun to set, then cover and cook until they are completely set, but the yolks are still runny. Sprinkle with parsley and serve.

Red Lentil Tikka Masala

218 calories per portion

Serves 4

FOR THE MASALA PASTE

2 teaspoons garam masala

2 teaspoons red pepper flakes

2 teaspoons smoked paprika

1 teaspoon cumin seeds, toasted and ground

1 teaspoon coriander seeds, toasted and ground

¾-inch-piece fresh ginger, peeled and grated

1 tablespoon peanut oil

2 tablespoons tomato paste

Salt and pepper

Handful of fresh coriander

FOR THE CURRY

1½ tablespoons vegetable oil

1 red onion, diced

2 tablespoons masala paste

1 clove garlic, crushed

1 (14-ounce) can diced tomatoes

1 cup vegetable stock

7 ounces red lentils, rinsed

7 ounces baby spinach leaves, washed

2 tablespoons low-fat plain yogurt

Pulse the masala paste ingredients in a food processor until smooth. Heat the oil in a large skillet, add the onion, and cook until softened, 3 to 4 minutes. Add the garlic and cook for another minute. Stir in the masala paste and cook to release flavors, then add the tomatoes and vegetable stock and bring to a boil. Add the lentils, reduce the heat, and simmer for 20 minutes. Remove from the heat and add the spinach leaves, allowing them to wilt in the warmth. If necessary, loosen with a little more hot stock and serve.

Madras Beef with Tomato and Red Onion Salad

319 calories per portion

Serves 4

    1 tablespoon vegetable oil
    1 onion, sliced
    2 cloves garlic, minced
    2 green bell peppers, seeded and sliced
    3 cardamom pods, bruised
    1 cinnamon stick
    4 red chiles, 2 seeded and finely chopped, 2 split
    2 teaspoons Madras curry powder, or to taste
    1 (14-ounce) can diced tomatoes
    1 tablespoon tomato paste
    1¾ pounds stewing or braising steak, trimmed of fat
        and cut into 1-inch cubes
    ½ teaspoon superfine sugar
    2 cups beef stock or boiling water and bouillon cube
    Cilantro, torn
    Salt and pepper

Preheat the oven to 325°F. Heat the oil in a casserole dish and sauté the onion, garlic, bell peppers, cardamom, cinnamon stick, and chopped red chiles for 5 to 7 minutes. Add the curry powder, stir, cook for another minute or two, and add the tomatoes and tomato paste. Cook over a medium heat for 5 minutes, stirring. Add the beef, halved red chiles, sugar, salt, and pepper, coat well, and cook for another 2 minutes. Add the stock, bring to a simmer, cover, and transfer to the oven. Cook for 1½ hours, or until the beef is tender. Serve with a salad of thinly sliced red onions and ripe tomatoes, with cilantro, and season with salt and black pepper.

Shrimp and Asparagus Stir-Fry
105 calories per portion

Serves 2

 1 teaspoon vegetable oil

 1 medium onion, sliced

 2 cloves garlic, crushed

 1 teaspoon ground ginger

 1 red bird's eye chile, seeded and finely chopped

 4 scallions, finely sliced on the diagonal

 1 lemongrass stalk, bruised

 2 Kaffir lime leaves

 3 tablespoons Thai fish sauce

 2 tablespoons boiling water

 ½ teaspoon palm sugar

12 raw jumbo shrimp

10 ounces asparagus, halved lengthwise and cut into
    1-inch pieces

Cilantro leaves, Thai basil leaves, and lime wedges
    to serve

Heat the oil in a wok, and stir-fry the onion, garlic, ginger, and chile until softened. Add the scallions, cook for another minute, then add the lemongrass, lime leaves, fish sauce, water, and sugar. Stir, then add the shrimp and asparagus. Cook on high heat for 3 minutes, or until the shrimp are pink and the asparagus is al dente. Remove the lemongrass. Serve with fresh cilantro, Thai basil, and a wedge of lime.

Field Mushrooms with Mozzarella, Pecorino, and Spinach
159 calories per portion

Serves 1

3.5 ounces baby spinach leaves, washed and wilted

½ teaspoon red pepper flakes

1 clove garlic, crushed

1 large or 2 medium field mushrooms, washed and
    dried

1.5 ounces low-fat mozzarella, shredded

2 teaspoons pecorino, grated or shaved

Fresh thyme leaves

Salt and pepper

Salad leaves to serve

Preheat the broiler to 400°F. Mix the spinach, red pepper flakes, and garlic in a small bowl and fill the mushroom cap. Place the mushroom on a grill rack and sprinkle with mozzarella. Scatter with pecorino and thyme leaves, season with salt and pepper, and grill for 7 to 10 minutes, or until the cheese has melted and the mushroom is cooked but still firm. Serve with dressed salad leaves.

And Six Tasty New Recipes to Try . . .

Dijon Chicken Dippers with Peas

281 calories per portion

Serves 2

    1 tablespoon Dijon mustard
    2 tablespoons low-fat plain yogurt
    1 teaspoon herbes de Provence
    Salt and pepper
    10 ounces mini chicken breast fillets
    7 ounces frozen peas
    6 mint leaves, finely chopped
    ½ red chile, seeded and finely chopped
    1 teaspoon butter

In a small bowl, combine the mustard, yogurt, and herbs. Season and add the chicken pieces, stirring to coat. Refrigerate until needed (up to 24 hours). Heat a grill pan and cook chicken until done, 8 to 10 minutes. Boil the peas and put half aside. Mash the remaining half with a fork, stir in the whole peas, adding the mint, chile, and butter. Stir, season well, and serve alongside the chicken.

Masala Salmon with Spiced Spinach
398 calories per portion

Serves 2
    ⅓ cup plain yogurt
    1 tablespoon masala paste
    1 teaspoon cumin seeds
    Salt and pepper
    2 salmon fillets (3.5 ounces each)

FOR THE SPICED SPINACH
    Cooking spray
    2 scallions, sliced
    1 clove garlic, crushed
    ½ teaspoon ground coriander
    Pinch cayenne pepper, or to taste
    ½ teaspoon garam masala
    2 cardamom pods, bruised
    10 ounces spinach leaves, washed
    Salt and pepper
    A squeeze of lemon

Heat the oven to 350°F. In a small bowl, combine the yogurt, masala paste, cumin seeds, salt, and pepper, then add the salmon fillets and coat well. Bake the salmon until opaque, about 15 minutes. Meanwhile, heat a pan and spray with oil. Sauté the scallion, garlic, and spices gently for 3 to 4 minutes until softened. Add the spinach, allowing it to wilt in the heat, adding a dash of water if necessary to prevent it sticking. Cook for 3 to 4 minutes, stirring gently. Remove from the heat, season, and add a squeeze of lemon. Serve alongside the warm baked salmon.

My Thai Mussels

470 calories per portion

Serves 2

¾-inch piece fresh ginger, peeled and julienned
1 lemongrass stalk, finely sliced
1 Kaffir lime leaf
1 red chile, seeded and finely sliced, or to taste
1 (14-ounce) can low-fat coconut milk
1 tablespoon Thai fish sauce
1 teaspoon sesame oil
2 pounds mussels, washed and debearded (discard any that aren't tightly closed)
Juice of ½ lime
Handful of fresh cilantro leaves
1 scallion, finely sliced
Lime wedges and red chile to serve

Place the ginger, lemongrass, lime leaf, and chile in a large pan with the coconut milk, fish sauce, and sesame oil. Bring to a boil and cook for 5 to 10 minutes. Add the mussels and cover the pan. Cook for 5 minutes, shaking occasionally, until the mussels are open and cooked (discard any that are shut). Add the lime juice, then serve in a large bowl, garnished with cilantro leaves, scallion, lime wedges, and a little more red chile, if desired.

Warm Eggplant Salad with Chickpeas and Halloumi

471 calories per portion

Serves 2

    1 tablespoon olive oil

    1 teaspoon ground cumin

    1 teaspoon paprika

    Salt and pepper

    1 to 2 eggplants (about 1 pound), cut into ¼-inch slices

    5 ounces low-fat halloumi cheese, sliced

    1 (14-ounce) can chickpeas, drained and rinsed

    7 ounces cherry tomatoes, halved

    Handful of flat-leaf parsley leaves, chopped

FOR THE DRESSING

    Handful of mint leaves, finely chopped

    ⅓ cup low-fat plain yogurt

    1 clove garlic, crushed

    2 teaspoons lemon juice

    Pinch of salt

Combine the dressing ingredients. In a separate small bowl, mix the oil, cumin, paprika, salt, and pepper and brush onto both sides of the eggplant slices. Heat a grill pan and cook the slices, turning once, until golden (about 5 minutes on each side), then set aside. Using the same pan, cook the halloumi, turning once, until lightly browned. Combine the chickpeas, tomatoes, and parsley with 2 teaspoons of the dressing. Top with the cooked eggplant and halloumi, drizzle with the remaining dressing, and add a final twist of pepper.

Baked Butternut Squash with Zucchini and Tomato
248 calories per portion, 290 calories with feta

Serves 2

    3 to 4 medium zucchini, cut on the diagonal into
        ¼-inch slices
    1 pound butternut squash, peeled and cubed
    1 vine of cherry tomatoes
    6 black olives (optional)
    1 head garlic, halved crosswise
    ½ lemon
    2 tablespoons olive oil
    Handful fresh thyme leaves
    Salt and pepper

Preheat the oven to 350°F. Place the prepared veggies in a small ovenproof dish, add the oil and lemon juice, adding the lemon husk to the dish. Season well. Bake for 25 minutes, until the garlic is softened and the veggies are beginning to caramelize. Perhaps serve with a sprinkle of feta (1 tablespoon per portion; add 42 calories). Alternatively, this works well as a side dish with any roasted or grilled meat.

Butterbean and Chorizo Hotpot
249 calories per portion

Serves 2

    1 ounce chorizo, finely chopped
    1 medium onion, peeled and finely diced
    2 cloves garlic, peeled and crushed
    1 (14-ounce) can butterbeans, drained and rinsed
    1 (14-ounce) can diced tomatoes
    1 tablespoon tomato paste
    1 teaspoon smoked paprika
    Pinch of sugar
    2 tablespoons water
    Salt and pepper
    Handful parsley, coarsely chopped, to serve

Heat a medium pan, add the chorizo, sauté to release its color and flavor. Add the onion and garlic, cooking gently until softened, about 5 minutes. Add the butterbeans, tomatoes, tomato paste, paprika, and sugar. Simmer for 15 minutes, stirring occasionally. Add 2 tablespoons of water, or a little more if the pan starts to look dry. Season and serve.

Straight to the Plate

I included some of these "fridge and cupboard" ideas in *FastDay Cookbook*, and they proved a popular way to get through supper on a fast day with minimum fuss. Not recipes so much as great flavor combinations, these trios can be grabbed from your fridge and kitchen cupboards on days when you just don't want to think too hard about food. Use lemon juice, balsamic vinegar (I like it in spray form) where necessary. Then just add a plate and a fork.

★ Shredded white cabbage + sliced red onion + hard-boiled egg (1 medium) **120 calories**

★ Smoked salmon (1.5 ounces) + hard-boiled egg (1 medium) + sliced fennel **180 calories**

★ Broad beans (3.5 ounces) + radicchio + pecorino (1.5 ounces) **196 calories**

★ Lean roast beef (3.5 ounces) + horseradish crème fraîche (1 tablespoon) + Boston lettuce **203 calories**

★ Chicken tikka pieces (5.5 ounces) + sliced beefsteak tomato + cucumber raita (2 tablespoons) **216 calories**

★ Avocado (half) + shrimp (5 ounces) + low-fat crème fraîche (1 tablespoon) **221 calories**

★ Prosciutto (4 slices) + melon + strawberries
228 calories

★ Mozzarella (1.5 ounces) + avocado (half) + 2 ripe
tomatoes **237 calories**

★ Baby spinach + prosciutto or ham (4 slices) +
Parmesan (1 tablespoon) **244 calories**

★ Low-fat hummus (3.5 ounces) + raw veggies +
jalapeños **246 calories**

★ Canned tuna (3.5 ounces) + cannellini beans
(3.5 ounces) + red onion **268 calories**

★ Cooked turkey breast (7 ounces) + arugula + pine
nuts (1 tablespoon) **269 calories**

★ Smoked chicken (5 ounces) + romaine lettuce +
cashews (1 tablespoon) **276 calories**

★ Blanched French beans + cooked jumbo shrimp
(5 ounces) + low-fat feta (3.5 ounces) **289 calories**

★ Roast beet (3.5 ounces) + low-fat halloumi
(3.5 ounces) + arugula **293 calories**

★ Low-fat feta (3.5 ounces) + hard-boiled egg
(1 medium) + red cabbage **295 calories**

★ Pilchards in olive oil (3.5 ounces) + cherry
  tomatoes + steamed broccoli florets **323 calories**

★ Smoked tilapia (3.5 ounces) + watercress + 4 plum
  tomatoes **354 calories**

★ Beef carpaccio (5 ounces) + toasted pine nuts
  (1 tablespoon) + arugula + Parmesan (1.5 ounces)
  404 calories

Fast Day Snacks

As we all know, there's little point in grazing on a fast
day—it would eliminate the point of the exercise. But some
people need a little lift, particularly in the early days when
their appetite is adjusting to the new routine. It's best to
avoid easy carbs and go instead for fresh, raw ingredients.
Have them prepped and handy in the fridge. Nuts, though
high in calories, are full of protein and good fats, and just a
few will help you feel full.

★ Licorice to chew, **0 calories**

★ Cherries, **33 calories for 2 ounces**

★ Blackberries, **25 calories for 3.5 ounces**

★ Strawberries, **30 calories for 8**

★ Miso soup packet, **32 calories**

★ Crudités: carrots sticks, celery stalks, cucumber sticks, raw pepper, watercress, radishes, cherry tomatoes, about **40 calories per serving**

★ Cottage cheese, **20 calories for 1 tablespoon**

★ Apple slices, including skin and core—add a squeeze of lemon juice, **60 calories**

★ Hard-boiled egg, **75–90 calories for 1** (depending on size)

★ Hummus, **56 calories for 1 tablespoon**

★ Handful of frozen grapes, **60 calories**

★ Pistachios, **60 calories for 10**

★ Almonds, **80 calories for 6**

★ Edamame, steamed and served warm with a little salt, **84 calories for 2 ounces**

★ Edam, **80 calories for 1 ounce**

★ Pumpkin and sunflower seeds, **90 calories for 1 tablespoon**

★ Air-popped popcorn, **93 calories for 3 cups**

The 5:2 Shopping List

Get in the habit of having fast-friendly food around—just enough to allow you to grab a quick meal when you're fasting and famished. Here's what you might have on hand. . . .

In the Fridge

Eggs
Low-fat hummus, low-fat plain yogurt, low-fat crème fraîche
Feta, cottage cheese, and low-fat mozzarella
Scallions
Chili peppers
Fresh herbs
Non-starchy veggies: cauliflower, broccoli, peppers, radishes, cherry tomatoes, celery, cucumber, mushrooms, lettuce, sugar snap peas, snow peas, salad leaves, and baby spinach
Carrots
Lemons
Strawberries, blueberries, apples

In the Cupboard

Canned tuna, in spring water
Cans of beans and chickpeas

Cans of tomatoes
Tomato paste
Garlic
Onions (red and white)
Mustard (Dijon and spicy yellow)
Vinegar (balsamic and white wine; try balsamic spritzer on
    salad)
Olive oil
Cooking spray
Spices, including cumin and coriander
Red pepper flakes
Nuts (unsalted are preferable)
Pickles (guindilla, jalapeños, cornichons, capers)
Bouillon cubes and miso paste
Sea salt and freshly ground black pepper
Unsweetened muesli
Sugar-free jelly
Shirataki noodles
Miso-soup packets

In the Freezer

Ginger—it is best grated from frozen
Broth, in empty (clean) soup and milk cartons
Soup—homemade or store-bought, in single portions
Blueberries, a cool little snack (strawberries don't freeze
    well)
Peas

Choosing the Right Frozen Dinner

If a frozen dinner is your only salvation during a busy week on the FastDiet, then take a few tips to help you make the right choices.

★ Look for meals with plants at their heart— accompanied by some "good" protein and slow-burn carbs. Avoid precooked pasta and potato dishes.

★ Check the portion size. Don't finish the box just because it tells you to. One FastDieter says she regularly uses a "Serves 2" meal to feed three.

★ Supplement your frozen dinner with easy-access fresh vegetables: grab half a bag of spinach leaves, a handful of arugula, Boston lettuce—whatever it takes to get your greens.

★ Soup can be a good option: again, look at the serving size and the calorie count

★ Even if you're eating in a hurry, try to do it sitting down, giving food your full attention.

Testimonials and Tweets

Mark Lovell, aged 44, Germany

Lost 31 pounds in 4 months (stable for over 13 months)

I never thought I would be writing a piece on dieting in any capacity. However, this comes from the heart as a very satisfied FastDiet convert.

In July 2013, after a dream vacation in the States, I topped the scales at an all-time high of 253 pounds and could not ignore the fact that I was overweight, despite claims that I supposedly "carried it well."

Looking back now, something must have gone "click" in my mind after watching Dr. Michael Mosley's excellent documentary, and I decided to take action. I was ready to try something different.

I plumped for Mondays and Thursdays as my fasting days and soon noticed a change in my habits. I learned that 600 calories is actually quite manageable with LOTS of salad and vegetables and that this is not a punishing diet.

I lost 37 pounds in four months and felt great. I learned that I didn't need to eat all the time and that in fact I could go a long time without eating. The beauty of the FastDiet for me is that I can still eat what I want on those nonfasting days. My favorite meal is still an Indian curry.

The biggest motivation is that the scales do not lie—this works. The FastDiet has now become a way of life, I am not fighting food anymore and I am enjoying life to the full. And not only do I feel hyperenergized, people have even told me I look a tad younger!

Mo Hayter, aged 66, Hampshire, England

Lost 24 pounds in 6 months

I started my FastDiet on 21 January 2015 when I read about it in the *Mail on Sunday*. I was about 42 pounds overweight with a BMI of 31 and all my attempts at losing weight had failed. I was really concerned on the first day that I'd faint or have some adverse effects, but I was fine and so I persevered. I lost 16 pounds in the first 2 months, after which the rate of my weight loss slowed down a lot but it is now steady. I've lost a total of 24 pounds and my BMI is down to 27. It's a way of life for me now so I intend to continue!

Before I started the diet, my blood pressure was very high, but it has been reduced significantly and I'm sure that's due to losing so much weight. My cholesterol was also very high, particularly the LDL (low-density lipoprotein), so I can't wait to see if it's improved (as Dr. Mosley's did) at my next checkup. One thing's for sure, I feel so much healthier and so happy that I've found such an easy way of losing weight. Not to mention my asthma has also improved.

Stella Minnet, aged 60, Swindon, England

Lost 42 pounds in 1 year

When I started the FastDiet, I weighed 176 pounds, the heaviest I had ever been. Even though I had been doing up to two or three exercise classes a week for the past three years, I'd steadily been putting on weight. I'm now down to 133 pounds, a loss of 42 pounds. I weigh less than I did when I got married at age 20! I love this way of life and am proud to have encouraged others to follow it too with great success. I still do several classes of exercises a week including body pump, circuits, and have started running again, which is so much easier at this weight! I'm now in size 12 jeans, down from a 16 this time last year.

The biggest change is the way I feel—being lighter on my feet, wearing smaller clothes, and taking pride in my achievement. And I really enjoy all the compliments!

Monica Michael, 27 years old, Cyprus

Lost 39 pounds in 5 months

I am a sufferer of PCOS (polycystic ovary syndrome) and the FastDiet has been AMAZING for me. After five months I'd already lost 39 pounds. I have also cured my insulin resistance and no longer need medication for it, and am no longer prediabetic. My PCOS is under control and my sugar levels have stabilized. My energy levels have soared and I eat a lot more healthily now, as I really think before I eat instead of just stuffing my face with processed junk foods. Buying *The FastBeach Diet* book was one of the best things I have ever done. I'm so glad I took the challenge to lose my last pounds before my holiday in Crete this year. I'm in better shape now than even before I had my three boys and am happy to wear my bikini for the first time in years!

Stephen Morris, 44 years old, Exmoor, England

Lost 42 pounds in 3 months

Over the years I have tried just about every diet going but have never really been able to stick with anything for more than ten days at a time. I'd get fed up when I woke up each morning, knowing that I faced yet another day of going without enjoyable food. To me, the word "diet" is really another word for "deprivation."

This is why the 5:2 has been such a revelation to me. I started doing the FastDiet around three months ago. The first fast day wasn't easy, but then again it wasn't as hard as I expected either. The second fast day was similar. After a week I'd dropped 5 pounds and I was happy. By the fourth week, the odd person began to notice a change, which was a great boost. All of a sudden the fasts were becoming quite easy, I was used to them. I wasn't at all bothered about a fast day approaching. In a strange way I started to look forward to them. I felt inspired and I was noticing things beyond the scales—an inch lost just about everywhere. One month became two and people really started to comment on my changing appearance. Suddenly it crept up on me, I'd been doing this for three months and had lost 42 pounds; all without really having to try too hard. This is so easy compared to anything else I've attempted. It really is a great way of eating as I still have a social life. A couple of days a week of discipline against five days of not worrying seems a very good deal to me.

So what's worth noting? Before starting the diet, I had a diabetes test and my levels were very high. My test a couple of weeks back showed that I no longer have anything to worry about. Energy-wise, I feel better than I have in years, no longer dreading exercise but enjoying it. I've walked the local cliff path where I live for years and I'm literally doing it in half the time it used to take me. Also, after years of terrible insomnia I'm starting to sleep better. I awake refreshed in the morning. Everyone notices the changes now! I'm getting into clothes I've not worn for years. On my nonfast days, I can go out and eat and drink what I want without guilt. But if I have a really heavy weekend I'll sometimes do an extra fast to compensate, but not always. I have just one rule: never ever quit a fast day. What keeps me going is knowing that tomorrow I can eat normally again.

Oh, and one other thing, I used to be totally dependent on sugar—not anymore. I can take it or leave it. If you'd said that to me three months ago, I'd have just laughed!

Debi Clayton, aged 49, Northants, England

Lost 49.5 pounds in 6 months

I downloaded *The FastDiet* around the New Year of 2014 because I hated how miserable my weight was making me. I rarely went out other than to go to work (I'm a secondary school teacher) and blamed the menopause for my considerable and rapid weight gain. I was making excuses in order not to walk our dogs so my husband did it because I got so tired, yet I was drinking a glass of wine most evenings to help me relax and fall asleep. Apart from HRT patches for the menopause, I was not on any other medication and I ate healthy food—or thought I did. The fact is that it became unhealthy due to the amount I was eating. I had no portion control. My porridge oats breakfast with water, yogurt, and berries was clocking up 700 calories!

After reading Michael and Mimi's book, I was convinced that I could manage the restricted calorie intake just twice a week. I was most impressed with the information about hunger not growing or worsening as time passed. I was very afraid of hunger! I started on the 13th January: my fast day consisted of black coffee (easy), sparkling mineral water with fresh lemon slices, two hard-boiled eggs, and a pear all consumed at lunchtime; then chicken salad and Diet Coke for dinner.

I was hungry but the pangs did not amount to more than a discomfort, which I soon found could be pacified with fluid and staying busy. The weight doesn't drop off in crazy amounts. Most weeks I lose .5 pound to 2 pounds but I've had fortnights of no loss, and then other weeks when I've lost 2.5 pounds.

I am now jogging with my younger dog! I can jump out of bed and go for a 6 a.m. run, I do my Zumba lessons, often with ankle weights and intensity level 3, I never consume wine to help me sleep. Actually, these days, I sleep like a baby regardless of my calorie intake. I feel alive and in charge of my life. I will not stop fasting just because I am a healthy weight. The benefits of feeling clearheaded, energized, and enjoying food tastes and textures is something I can't give up. I have played about with my fasting methods and now on a fast day prefer to consume fluids and save my calorie allowance in order to enjoy one substantial meal.

Dan Smith, aged 40, Worcestershire, England

Lost 36 pounds in 1 year

In November 2012, I was two months from my fortieth birthday and 177 pounds (the heaviest I've ever been) and felt that, if I was going to effect a positive change in my life, it was now or never.

I was inspired to try the FastDiet by two friends who achieved amazing results following the BBC program in 2012. I needed to do something to lose weight, look and feel better. The FastDiet made sense and appeared sustainable as a way of life rather than a short-term fix.

The fast days were challenging at first, until I realized

that coping with hunger is actually quite easy. I changed my relationship with food, my awareness of my diet and body, giving me control over my weight. By July 2013, I was 149 pounds, the only downside being the need for new, smaller clothes! I have far more energy than before, have had no colds or illness, and have inspired at least three others to begin their own FastDiet.

I feel great and genuinely in the best shape I've ever been. Thank you, Michael Mosley et al.—you have changed a lot of lives for the better.

Eleri Roberts, aged 25, Cumbria, England

Lost 14 pounds in 6 months

I started the FastDiet after watching the documentary and then reading the book. It sounded like just what I needed. I wasn't hugely overweight. I just had a few extra pounds I wanted to lose to get back into shape. Other diets put me off; the thought of giving up on treats indefinitely sounded depressing and unrealistic, so I gave 5:2 a try.

The first few fast days were hard, I thought about food *all* day and fantasized about my next nonfast day. However, at the end of just one week I felt amazing, energized, clean, and healthy.

I soon got into a routine of saving all 500 calories for a satisfying evening meal and began to really look forward to the clean and healthy feeling gained from a fast day.

In just a couple of weeks I noticed I was actually unable

to eat three full meals on my five diet-free days and no longer craved so many naughty treats. Overall, in six months I have lost over 14 pounds and reached my target weight easily. Amazing considering I have drunk wine, eaten plenty of chocolate and takeout, and had big breakfasts!

I would recommend the 5:2 to anyone; it is not just a diet, but a realistic and manageable lifestyle change.

Britt Warg, aged 58, Swindon, England

Lost 15 pounds, and has been stable for 2 years

I started the FastDiet just a few days after Michael Mosley's first BBC broadcast and have been sticking to it ever since, apart from a few "breaks." I have fasted two days a week—and sometimes three.

The diet makes me feel good, happier with myself, and more energetic. I have never found it hard to keep it up but at certain times, "life" has got in the way. One such period was when my mom back in Sweden was dying from Alzheimer's and I traveled back and forth over several months. I also find it difficult to turn down friends' dinner requests, especially if I am the only one invited and they have made an effort to cook.

Before going on a sun-and-sea holiday in May of 2015, I made an extra effort to lose weight and managed to lose 15 pounds in about three months. This was achieved by sticking to the same diet and greatly increasing the number of regular walks I was taking. I work from home and my daily routine involves a lot of writing. I also stand up while working a lot more and sometimes do "silly" leg and arm movements—when nobody is watching! In shops, I take the stairs instead of escalators. I walk to the shops, instead of driving or taking the bus. Every little bit helps!

Another observation: I now need less of my thyroxine tablets. I used to take 150 mg but this was reduced to 125 mg a year ago and more recently has been further reduced to 100 mg. High cholesterol sadly runs in my family, but my levels have gone down. Also, I do a voluntary, yearly "life screening," to check for carotid artery disease, atrial fibrillation, abdominal aortic aneurysm, and peripheral arterial disease. Two years ago, there was a mild plaque buildup in my right carotid artery, but this year, it was back to normal.

Tweets

@iamdougroper

Thrilled to have lost a stone following @TheFastDietBook & finding 5:2 combined with exercise is good for general physical/mental health! :)

@LovellLowdown

Vastly improved my pollen allergies. Used to suffer horribly #thefastdiet

@Roband68

2 weeks into the fastdiet and ¾ inch off the waistline and 6.5 pounds lost!!!

@mahgnilloc

16 months on fastdiet and off asthma meds for the last 4 months #thefastdiet #notjustadiet

@therealjuicybug

Been a 5:2 fan for 14 months & been off medication for gastric reflux problems for 12 months now. #eatclean #fastdiet

@theothersilvia

I used to be your biggest fan, but with your diet and recipes I lost 39 pounds, so I guess I'm a small one now.

@tracygreen72

Lost 6 pounds in total up to now on @TheFastDietBook (in 3 weeks and 2 days). Why didn't I discover this diet years ago! @DrMichaelMosley #legend

@ds14

Started in November 12, went from 177 to current weight of 141. Fitter, faster, and happier than when I was 17. Now 40!

@Suethebold

@TheFastDietBook @mimispencer1 regained my confidence #nothingelseworked

@alert_bri

After 4 months on 5:2, agree with your doc assessment . . . this could change the world. Your book should fuel the revolution.

Calorie Counter

FOOD	SERVING SIZE	CALORIES PER SERVING
PROTEIN		
Almonds	6	80
Bacon, lean	1 oz./1 slice	70
Chicken breast, fat removed	4 oz./1 medium	175
Chicken thigh, fat removed	3 oz./1 medium	170
Egg	1 large	90
Egg	1 medium	80
Ham, lean	1½ oz./1 slice	60
Roast beef, fat removed	1¼ oz./1 slice	51
Salmon, fresh fillet	5 oz./1 fillet	275
Salmon, smoked	2 oz.	66
Shrimp, peeled	2 oz./10 large	58
Sirloin steak, fat removed	5 oz.	188
Tilapia, fresh fillet	6 oz.	320

FOOD	SERVING SIZE	CALORIES PER SERVING
Tilapia, smoked	3½ oz.	202
Tofu	5¼ oz.	96
Trout fillet, smoked	1¾ oz.	75
Tuna, canned in oil	2¾ oz.	101
Tuna, canned in spring water	2¾ oz.	76
Tuna steak	5 oz./1 fillet	225
Turkey breast, cooked	1¼ oz./1 slice	39
White fish fillet	6¼ oz./1 fillet	175
DAIRY		
Cheddar cheese, low-fat	1¾ oz.	165
Cottage cheese, low-fat	1¾ oz./ 1 tablespoon	20
Cream cheese, low-fat	1¼ oz./ 1 tablespoon	55
Crème fraîche, low-fat	¾ oz./ 1 tablespoon	50
Edam	1¾ oz.	158
Feta	1¾ oz.	85
Goat cheese (log)	1¾ oz.	161
Milk, 1%	4 oz.	50
Milk, 2%	4 oz.	60
Milk, almond (unsweetened)	4 oz.	20
Milk, rice	4 oz.	47
Milk, skim	4 oz.	43
Milk, soy (unsweetened)	4 oz.	31
Mozzarella, low-fat	2 oz.	140
Parmesan, grated	¼ oz./ 1 tablespoon	28

FOOD	SERVING SIZE	CALORIES PER SERVING
Yogurt, low-fat plain yogurt	¾ oz./1 tablespoon	15
CARBS		
Basmati rice, brown, cooked (2 oz. uncooked)	5¼ oz.	189
Bran flakes	1¾ oz.	144
Bread, white	1 medium slice	96
Bread, whole-wheat	1 medium slice	88
Bulgur, cooked	5¼ oz.	165
Couscous, cooked	3½ oz.	152
Egg noodles, cooked	5¼ oz.	198
Muesli, fruit and nut	1¾ oz.	177
Noodles, rice, cooked	5¼ oz.	222
Noodles, Shirataki	7 oz.	4
Oatmeal, old-fashioned rolled	1½ oz.	155
Potatoes, cooked or baked	8½ oz./ 1 medium	233
Potatoes, new, boiled or steamed	7 oz.	150
Quinoa, cooked	3¾ oz.	132
Spaghetti, cooked (3½ oz. uncooked)	8¼ oz.	371
Spaghetti, whole-wheat, cooked (3½ oz. uncooked)	8½ oz.	310
Tortilla, flour	1⅓ oz./1 tortilla	150
Tortilla, whole-wheat	1⅓ oz./1 tortilla	144
FATS		
Butter	¼ oz./ 1 teaspoon	52
Margarine	1 teaspoon	34

FOOD	SERVING SIZE	CALORIES PER SERVING
Olive oil	1 teaspoon	40
Vegetable oil	1 teaspoon	40
VEGETABLES		
Arugula	2 oz.	20
Asparagus	3½ oz./ 5 medium	33
Avocado	½ medium	120
Baby corn	3 oz.	22
Baked beans, low-salt and sugar	7¼ oz./½ can	145
Bell pepper, red	5½ oz./ 1 medium	50
Broccoli	3½ oz.	34
Butterbeans, cooked	4¼ oz.	126
Cabbage, green	8½ oz.	63
Cabbage, white	5 oz./ ¼ medium head	40
Carrot	4¼ oz./2 small	45
Cauliflower	5 oz.	37
Celery	1¾ oz./ 1 medium stalk	8
Celery root	7 oz./¼ bulb	84
Cherry tomatoes	4 oz./ 10 tomatoes	20
Chickpeas, cooked	4¼ oz.	132
Corn, frozen	2¾ oz.	78
Corn on the cob	4 oz./1 ear	150
Cucumber	3½ oz./ ¼ medium	17
Eggplant	4½ oz.	25

FOOD	SERVING SIZE	CALORIES PER SERVING
Fennel bulb	7 oz.	62
French green beans	1¾ oz.	16
French green lentils	3¾ oz./½ can	86
Garlic	1 clove	3
Kidney beans, cooked	4½ oz.	180
Leek	3½ oz./1 large	25
Lettuce	3¾ oz.	19
Mushrooms, button	2½ oz.	17
Mushroom, portobello	3½ oz./ 1 medium	15
Olives, black or green	½ oz./5 medium	40
Onion	5¾ oz./ 1 medium	66
Peas, frozen	2¾ oz.	52
Snow peas	3½ oz.	18
Spinach, fresh	3½ oz.	23
Sugar snap peas	1¾ oz.	43
Tomatoes, canned	7 oz.	44
Tomatoes, fresh	7 oz./2 medium	36
Watercress	2 oz.	12
Zucchini	5 oz./1 medium	33

FRUIT

Apple	3½ oz./1 small	50
Apricots	3 oz./2 medium	35
Apricots, dried	1 oz./5 small	72
Banana	4 oz./1 medium	95
Blueberries	2 oz./ 20 blueberries	35

FOOD	SERVING SIZE	CALORIES PER SERVING
Cantaloupe	7¾ oz./1 medium wedge	53
Cherries	3⅓ oz./ 10 cherries	49
Dates	¾ oz./3 pitted	70
Fig	1¾ oz./ 1 medium	24
Fruit compote	3½ oz.	65–80
Grapefruit	5 oz./½ medium	52
Grapes	2¼ oz./ 10 grapes	43
Honeydew melon	4 oz./1 medium wedge	45
Kiwi fruit	2 oz./1 medium	42
Lemon juice	½ lemon	6
Lime juice	½ lime	2
Orange	5½ oz./ 1 medium	70
Pear	6½ oz./ 1 medium	94
Plum	2 oz./1 medium	24
Raisins	½ oz.	44
Raspberries	2 oz./20–25 raspberries	32
Strawberries	3½ oz./ 8 large	30
Tangerine	2¾ oz./ 1 medium	45
Watermelon	11 oz./ 1 large wedge	105

Part Two

FastExercise

Introduction
to FastExercise

AS A MEDICALLY TRAINED JOURNALIST I FRE-quently come across claims that seem too good to be true and often are. Occasionally, after dig-ging around, I reconsider my original position, acknowledge that what might appear at first to be outra-geous could have something in it. As the economist John Maynard Keynes once said, "When the facts change, I change my mind."

This happened to me when, in early 2012, I first heard about intermittent fasting. My initial reaction was skepti-cism. I assumed it would turn out to be some variation on "detoxing" or other largely discredited views of how the body works. Nonetheless I decided to find out more as I'd recently discovered that I was a borderline diabetic with too much visceral fat (the fat that lies inside your abdomen). My father had died from a diabetes-related illness and I could see myself going down the same road.

So I set out to examine the claim that you can lose weight and get health benefits, particularly improvements in your insulin, by changing your pattern of eating. I soon came across research done in the United States and the United Kingdom which pointed to rapid fat loss and other benefits that would come from cutting my calories, not every day, but just a few days a week.

As I looked deeper I discovered intermittent fasting was backed by a significant body of animal and human research. I spoke to many eminent experts, tested the claims on myself, and made a documentary for the BBC. Then, in January 2013, I wrote a book with Mimi Spencer, *The FastDiet*, which summarized all this research into what we called a 5:2 diet (eat normally five days a week, cut your calories for two). Using this method, I lost over 20 pounds of fat and my blood glucose returned to a normal level. Although this was just my experience (and personal anecdotes make poor science) it was in line with a number of clinical studies done on different forms of intermittent fasting.

We still don't know the ideal pattern for intermittent fasting, the true long-term benefits, or the potential pitfalls, but since the book was published many thousands of people have followed the 5:2 regime, lost weight, and contacted me to say how easy it is. And I'm pleased to say new studies are underway.

While writing *The FastDiet*, one of the areas I touched on—but only briefly—was exercise. Diet and exercise are complementary, they go together like Fred Astaire and Ginger Rogers, like Batman and Robin. And, as we will see, there are interesting parallels in the way science is transforming the way we think about both.

Before making the film on fasting, I had come across a rapidly developing new area of exercise research called high-intensity interval training (HIIT), also known as HIT (high-intensity training).

One of the pioneers of this radically different approach to exercise is Jamie Timmons, Professor of Systems Biology at Loughborough University. Loughborough is home to the Centre for Olympic Studies and Research and has one of the leading sports research departments in the United Kingdom.

When we met, Jamie made what I thought was an outrageous, almost unbelievable claim. He said that I could get many of the more important benefits of exercise from just three minutes of intense exercise a week. He said that if I was prepared to give it a go he was confident that in just four weeks I would see significant changes in my biochemistry. It seemed wildly unlikely but also immensely intriguing. So I got myself properly tested and then I went for it. The results, which I discuss on page 273, were a revelation.

Since I had an initial conversation with Jamie back in 2011, research on HIT has exploded, with new findings coming out all the time. There has been a wealth of new studies providing mounting evidence that you really can get many of the same benefits from short bursts of intense effort as you can from following the more traditional approach, or perhaps even more. Benefits which include:

★ Improved aerobic fitness and endurance

★ Reduced body fat

★ Increased upper and lower body strength

★ Improved insulin sensitivity

These research findings form the basis of what I've called FastExercise, a practical and enjoyable way to get the maximal benefits in the minimal time.

My coauthor, leading sports journalist and coach Peta Bee, has spent her career investigating the claims of the sport and fitness industry. Unlike me she loves exercise. She's provided invaluable experience which has helped turn theory into practice.

The Dynamo and the Slob

MICHAEL'S MOTIVATION

Peta and I approach exercise from very different perspectives. She is fantastically sporty and has been from an early age. She runs marathons for fun and adores a good, hard workout. She has spent the last twenty years thinking, writing, and training others to share her passion.

I, on the other hand, don't like exercise. I don't get a high from working out or pushing myself; instead I share the views of astronaut Neil Armstrong who once said, "I believe that every human has a finite amount of heartbeats. I don't intend to waste any of mine running around doing exercises." Or the actor Peter O'Toole who claimed, "The only exercise I take is walking behind the coffins of friends who took exercise."

All right, that is an exaggeration. Now aged 56, I see the need and I appreciate the value of being active. I also fully embrace the idea that we are born to move. When I was at medical school I played quite a lot of sports, went for runs, and swam. Then I started working and could no longer find the time.

Don't get me wrong; I am not a complete slob. I love skiing, enjoy walks, relish swimming in the sea, and like being active. I don't actually think of any of these as "exercise," something you do because you think you should.

Exercise for me means the gym. It means going for long runs even when it is wet and cold, or trudging away on the treadmill; it is hours getting sweaty on an exercise bike or lifting heavy weights, followed by those incredulous moments when you step on the weighing scales and discover that you have hardly shifted a pound. For me, exercise is there to be endured, done because you have to, not because you want to.

If I am going to exercise I want it to be short, sharp, easy to do, and soon over. This, along with the science, is what first attracted me to HIT. Peta, as you might expect, came to HIT for different reasons.

PETA'S MOTIVATION

Unlike Michael, I love exercise and the way it makes me feel. I enjoy testing my own endurance and strength and relish the fatigue that comes with being absolutely physically spent.

My love affair with exercise started when I took up athletics at primary school—a start which eventually saw me run for Wales in my teens and early twenties. My passion for understanding how the body responds to intense effort, how it is repeatedly able to push itself to new limits, led me to study sports science at university. It was during that time that I gained a grounding in the basic principles of physiology and biomechanics and this cemented my view of fitness and how to attain it. Fitness eventually became the prime focus of my career as a journalist, and for the past twenty years I have written about sports science and fitness and their impact on health and longevity.

As for HIT, in all my many years of exercising and studying the practice of exercise, I have found nothing that comes close to producing the physical and mental rewards of it. I suppose in some ways I am the living embodiment of a lifelong FastExerciser—not that I realized it until recently. My induction into the concept of intense bursts of effort with short bouts of recovery occurred when I first started athletics training. Several times a week I would sprint-jog, sprint-jog my way around the track—a practice I have kept up with varying degrees of effort to this day as I race up hills, around alternate edges of a football pitch, between lampposts, and along lines of trees.

Now, at 45, a busy, working mom, I no longer have the time or, to be honest, the inclination to spend more than an hour a day working out. Yes, I want to offset middle-age weight gain, to feel good, and, of course, look as good as I can. And I want a body that performs well. But I want it fast. And that, in short, is the greatest appeal of HIT for me. If you want to discover a way to get fit quickly, with minimal time commitment, read on.

The role of science is to question. It is by doing experiments that traditional thinking is challenged and sometimes overthrown. So, where does that leave widely held exercise beliefs? Claims such as:

★ To get maximum benefit you should do lots of moderate-intensity exercise

★ If you exercise you will lose weight

★ You should always do lengthy warm-ups before exercising

★ Stretching before exercise will improve your performance and reduce your risk of injury

★ We all get benefit from doing exercise

In Part Two we take a good, hard look at these and other claims. In the first part, Michael looks at the history and science of HIT, and his own attempts to put theory into practice. In the second part, Peta has put together a range of evidence-based FastExercise workouts, along with practical advice and tips on how to integrate HIT into your life.

We want you to be as skeptical about our conclusions as we are about others'. We have included numerous references to the scientific literature that we have drawn on so that you can make your own judgments. These studies can be easily accessed through an Internet search; most are free in their entirety; all are available as abstracts.

We owe an enormous debt of gratitude to the numerous scientists and volunteers who have devoted their time and their bodies to uncovering the truths about exercise and who have put themselves through a range of strenuous routines in the hope of discovering the optimal ways to work out.

No one size will fit all but we hope this book will give you the information you need to create an effective and enjoyable exercise regime that works for you.

This is a book for those who, like Michael, don't enjoy exercise but who want to keep down the fat and stay healthy in the most effective, time-efficient way. It is for those, like Peta, who love exercise and want to get the most from it. It is also for those who are simply curious about themselves and who like having their preconceptions challenged. Enjoy.

CHAPTER FOUR

The Truth About Exercise

EVEN ON A DAY WHEN IT'S COLD AND GRAY OUTSIDE and the last thing you want to do is pull on your trainers, there are good reasons for getting up and going out. Regular exercise is a powerful antiaging medicine, providing a wide range of health and psychological benefits, from strengthening your bones to improving your brain, from reducing cancer risk to boosting your mood. You might even look better on the beach.

Yet exercise, like diet, is an area that is swathed in popular misconceptions. There is a huge gap between what sports scientists know about exercise and what is actually done in gyms and public parks. In recent years new studies have overturned much of what we once thought was well established.

Based on the latest research, Part Two of this book will reveal, among other things:

★ How to get fit in a few minutes a day

★ Why some people get so much more benefit from exercise than others

★ Why high-volume, low-intensity exercise like jogging rarely leads to weight loss

This last claim is in many ways the most surprising and disheartening. After all, the main reason why many of us take up jogging or join a gym is because we believe it will help us shed the pounds. Burn calories, lose weight.

If only things were so simple. Study after study has shown that conventional, low-intensity exercise like jogging or swimming rarely leads to weight loss. If you want to lose fat then intensity is the key.

So What Are the Measurable Benefits of Exercise?

Exercise and Longevity

One of the things we'd all expect regular exercise would lead to is a longer, healthier life. But how active do you need to be and what sort of exercise should you be doing?

Thanks to a recent review of 22 separate studies[1] which followed nearly a million people from Europe, North America, East Asia, and Australasia, we know that a couch potato who gets off the sofa and starts doing around 2.5

hours of moderate activity a week (walking, cycling, jogging, swimming) can expect to reduce their mortality risk by around 19%.

That sounds pretty impressive and it is the sort of figure bandied around by experts in the hope that it will encourage people to move more. The trouble is, it doesn't. Despite numerous public health campaigns, most Europeans and North Americans don't come close to doing 2.5 hours of moderate activity a week. Fewer than 20% of us do anything like the recommended levels.

There are many barriers to getting more active (lack of time is the commonest excuse), but I also think the way in which the benefits of exercise are presented is not particularly compelling or convincing.

"Mortality risk," for example, is a concept that is difficult to grasp and not a great motivator. To get a better grip on what "mortality risk" means I asked a statistician friend to try and explain this finding in a more comprehensible way.

After grinding the numbers he concluded that if you are bone idle and start doing about twenty minutes of exercise a day then that will add about 2.2 years to your life expectancy.

Adding 2.2 years to life expectancy sounds reasonable, but if to get this return I have to exercise 2.5 hours a week and I don't particularly enjoy it, is that really a good investment of my time? And if I do more will I get more benefit?

Fortunately, there is another, more interesting way of looking at this sort of data. It is called "Microlives," and it is the brainchild of Professor David Spiegelhalter of Cambridge

University. It is a brave attempt to turn complex studies into understandable facts.

What Professor Spiegelhalter realized is that once you hit your midtwenties you can expect to live around 57 more years. Fifty-seven years conveniently translates into half a million hours, or a million 30-minute chunks of life. These 30-minute chunks he calls microlives.

Based on this idea, Professor Spiegelhalter went through lots of studies[2] and started calculating the number of microlives you win or lose by doing a range of different activities. Smoking 20 cigarettes a day, for example, shortens your life expectancy by around eight years. This means that every pack of cigarettes you smoke will reduce your life by around 10 microlives or about five hours.

On the other hand, each portion of fruit and vegetables you eat adds just under one microlife, so if you eat the recommended five portions a day you should get an extra four years of life, mainly because of your reduced risk of heart disease.

I was pleased to see that, according to the *New England Journal of Medicine*, drinking a moderate amount of coffee is good for you. In fact, it turns out that drinking 2–3 cups of coffee a day (and it doesn't seem to matter much whether it is caffeinated or not) will add one microlife—possibly thanks to the flavonoids in it which have an antioxidant effect. This means that the two cups of coffee I drink every morning not only make me sharper and cheerier afterwards, they are time well spent.

If I spend ten minutes drinking coffee and each time I

have a cup I am adding around 30 minutes to my life, then that looks like a real bargain. (Unfortunately, if you go much beyond three cups a day the benefits begin to fade.)

So how well does exercise compare with drinking coffee or eating vegetables? Pretty well, at least to start with. If you are a slob and start exercising for twenty minutes a day that will buy you two microlives—an extra hour of life.

But the benefits of doing more exercise, at least in terms of life expectancy, then drop off dramatically. This is not a linear relationship. If you decide to exercise for an hour a day this will not add six microlives. The extra 40 minutes of exercise will, at most, only get you 1 extra microlife.

In other words, after the first twenty minutes, the next twenty minutes of moderate exercise you do will only buy you an extra fifteen minutes of life. If, like me, you don't enjoy those twenty minutes it begins to look like a rather bad investment.

This is all a bit artificial because there are clearly costs and benefits to be had that are not reflected in mortality statistics. If I smoke 20 cigarettes a day, for example, I am not only going to die younger, I am probably going to spend the last few decades of my life coughing, wheezing, and generally feeling wretched. Similarly, if I exercise regularly I am likely to be more active, alert, and to take fewer drugs in old age. In truth, most of us know which we would prefer.

How Exercise Benefits Your Brain

I am very fond of my brain so I was particularly encouraged when I came across a number of studies that point out how good exercise is, not just for the body, but also for the brain.

In a study done at the University of Illinois,[3] they took 59 healthy but sedentary volunteers, aged 60–79, and randomly allocated them to one of two programs: either aerobic training or "toning and stretching" exercises done for six months. Before and after the volunteers did these exercises, they had scans to measure the size of their brains.

The results were extremely interesting: there were significant increases in the brain volume of those doing the fitness training, but not of those who just did the stretching and toning.

One reason why this happens may be because exercise leads to the release of all sorts of proteins in the brain, including BDNF (brain-derived neurotrophic factor). This protein helps protect existing brain cells and encourages the development of new ones.

So you get a bigger brain, but also one that is probably better protected against dementia.

In another intriguing study,[4] researchers followed 20,000 men and women who had had their baseline fitness measured between 1971 and 2009. During that time, 1,659 of them developed dementia. Scarily, the ones who were the least fit were almost twice as likely to succumb to dementia as those who were most fit.

This was not an exercise intervention study, so we do not know if embarking on a fitness program will actually make a difference. But it seems plausible.

So Much for the Benefits. What Are the Risks?

The evidence is strong that moving is much better than not moving; and, if you are like Peta and enjoy exercise for its own sake, then working out is time well spent, whatever the tangible health benefits. However, it is worth pointing out that recent studies suggest that more is not necessarily better.

We know, for example, that excessive exercise can lead to long-term damage of your joints.

My father, who was a keen rugby player when he was young, spent the last decade of his life in a lot of pain in his knees as a result of injuries which occurred when he was in his twenties. We know that arthritis of the lower joints (particularly knees) is far more common in footballers and some athletes than in the normal population, and a study of former PE teachers in Sweden turned up some pretty disturbing findings.

In a study published in the *Journal of Occupational and Environmental Health*,[5] researchers tracked down more than 500 men and women who had qualified from the Gymnastiska Centralinstitutet, a training college for PE teachers in

Sweden, between 1957 and 1965. The subjects were, at the time of the study, mainly in their late fifties. The researchers then chose a matched group of people from the general Swedish population and did a comparison.

What they found was that the former PE teachers had far higher rates of arthritis of the knee and hip than the matched group of contemporaries. Despite being slimmer and more health conscious, they were three times more likely to have arthritis in the knees than people from the general population. In fact, their problems were so severe that only 20% were still working as PE teachers, and in a number of cases their joints had needed replacement surgery.

Joint problems are common in impact sports, but oddly enough this is not the case among runners. If anything, running seems to be protective. The risk to runners who overdo it seems to be more from damage to the heart than to the joints.

An editorial published in the June 2013 edition of the *Journal of Applied Physiology*[6] pointed out that half of serious rowers and marathon runners showed early signs of fibrosis in their hearts. Fibrosis, a form of scarring, can lead to irregular heartbeats which in turn can lead to more significant problems.

Before you get too worried I should stress that the men who were studied had undergone immense amounts of training, far more than the average distance runner, and this damage may be reversible, at least it is in rats.

Nonetheless, some cardiologists who study the impact of exercise are concerned about the effects of extreme endurance sports on the heart. The authors of this review (who were both once keen long-distance runners) point out that the very first marathon runner, Phidippides, a courier who ran the 26.2 miles from Marathon to Athens to announce news of a Greek victory, dropped dead on arrival.

The odds of that happening to a modern-day marathon runner are small, but as these cardiologists point out, "chronic extreme exercise seems to cause wear and tear on the heart."

Research from Denmark has also raised a few alarms about jogging too far and too fast.[7]

In 1975 a team in Copenhagen began following a group of 20,000 Danes aged between 20 and 93. Some did regular exercise, most did not. At the start of the study and throughout the years that followed, the volunteers kept a record of how much jogging they did, how far, and how intensely. Over the course of the last 37 years more than 10,000 of the people in the study have died.

By comparing death rates between joggers and nonjoggers, the researchers were able to show that jogging can add around four years to your life, which is in line with studies I mentioned earlier. This finding, when it was published, was widely reported. What was less covered was the finding that you seem to get the maximum benefits if you don't do too much.

The ideal, at least based on this study, is to jog for 30–50 minutes, three days a week, at a pace at which you feel "a little breathless but not very breathless." You can still chat but probably not sing. Recovery days are important, which is why it is better to jog three times a week than twenty minutes every day.

The sting in the tail is that beyond a certain point doing more exercise may be counterproductive. When the researchers looked at the data in detail they concluded that "these results showed a tendency of a U-shaped relation to mortality risk." In other words, doing some running is better than sitting on the sofa, but doing lots of running may not be better than doing a moderate amount.

We don't know at what point "a lot" becomes "too much" but if you are exercising for more than an hour a day you are probably doing it for reasons other than optimizing your health.

How Can You Tell If Exercise Is Doing You Any Good?

It's all very well having big studies showing the average improvements in mortality that can be expected from doing different levels of exercise, but most of us want advice that is more personal.

How do you know if a new exercise regime is improving your health, extending *your* life? The obvious measure, standing on the weighing scales, is not going to be particularly revealing—not only because the scales are unlikely to move much but because changes in weight are not the best predictor of future benefits (see page 243).

So what are the changes that matter? Increased strength and flexibility are important, and we include a list at the back of the book of the sort of things you might want to measure before starting an exercise regime, but two of the most important measures are aerobic fitness and glucose tolerance.

Aerobic Fitness

Aerobic fitness refers to your endurance or ability to keep going while doing something like jogging or running. It is a measure of how strong your heart and lungs are and how well they respond to the stresses placed upon them.

The most widely accepted way of measuring aerobic fitness is VO2 max. This is the maximum amount of oxygen that your body can use while you are doing intense exercise. Another way of looking at it is that VO2 max is a measure of how good your heart and lungs are at getting oxygen into and around your body—how strong your engine is.

VO2 max is not just a measure of how fit you are, but a powerful predictor of future health. We worry about cholesterol, alcohol, being overweight. Yet none of these matter anything like as much as your VO2 max. People with good levels of aerobic fitness are much less likely to get heart disease, cancer, diabetes, or become demented.

As we'll see in later chapters, most people's VO2 max rises quite sharply in response to exercise, particularly if the exercise is intense. The best way to get your aerobic fitness measured is in a lab or gym, but there are also ways to do it yourself, which we outline at the back of the book.

Glucose Tolerance

In 1922 three scientists called Banting, Best, and Collip went into a ward full of comatose and dying children. They injected each child with a substance recently extracted from the pancreas of a calf fetus. Before they had reached the last child the first children were already coming out of their comas. Their parents, who had been told nothing could be done, wept in shocked delight. It was a glorious moment in the long history of medicine, a miracle. The substance they had injected was insulin.

The reason those children were in comas was because they had Type 1 diabetes. They were dying because their bodies could no longer produce enough insulin. As a result their blood sugar levels had risen out of control.

Prior to the identification, extraction, and purification of insulin there was little that could be done for children with Type 1 diabetes. They became intensely hungry and thirsty before slipping into a coma and dying. The only treatment that appeared to make any difference was severe calorie restriction.

The villain was glucose. Glucose is an essential part of our lives, the main fuel that our cells use for energy. But glucose is also toxic. Persistently high levels are associated with all sorts of unpleasant consequences, ranging from increased risk of diabetes, blindness, kidney failure, and heart disease to amputation, cancer, dementia, and death.

Fortunately, most of us have a pancreas that will respond to a surge in glucose by pumping out insulin. Insulin is a sugar controller; it aids the extraction of glucose from blood and then stores it in places like your liver or muscles in a stable form called glycogen, to be used if and when it is needed.

What is less commonly known is that insulin is also a fat controller. It inhibits lipolysis, the release of stored body fat. At the same time, it forces fat cells to take up and store fat from your blood. High levels of insulin lead to increased fat storage, low levels to fat depletion.

The trouble with a Western diet, drenched in fat and sugary, carbohydrate-rich foods and drinks, is that it forces your pancreas to pump out ever increasing quantities of insulin. Up to a point this magnificent organ will cope, but ultimately it will simply give up. You are now a diabetic.

Rates of diabetes worldwide have increased tenfold in the last decade and there are now at least 285 million diabetics, most of them Type 2. Unlike Type 1, which normally occurs in childhood, Type 2 is largely a result of being overweight and inactive. By 2030 at least 500 million people are expected to be diagnosed as diabetic, with the same number undiagnosed.

Why Blood Sugar Levels Matter to Everyone, Not Just Diabetics

Though we don't know it, many of us have persistently high levels of both glucose and insulin which, while they are not in the diabetic range, are nonetheless an indicator of future problems.

Excess glucose in the blood—that is, glucose which has not been taken up by our cells—binds to body proteins (a process called glycation), damaging arteries and nerves. It also makes us look older. In a recent study[8] 600 men and women had their blood glucose levels measured and then, on the basis of their photos, had their age estimated. Diabetics and those with higher blood sugar levels were perceived as being significantly older than they were. This is probably because excess glucose attacks collagen and elastin, proteins that help make skin look supple and youthful.

One of the more important measures of your biological fitness is how swiftly and effortlessly your body is able to get your blood glucose back down to safe levels. See the back of the book for more details.

Although most forms of exercise will improve your aerobic and metabolic fitness, intensity seems to be particularly important for improving both. Intensity also matters when it comes to weight loss.

The Weight-Loss Fallacy—Why Long and Slow Is Not the Way to Go

One of the main reasons we take up exercise is because we have been led to believe that it will help us lose weight. We stand on the scales, gulp, and join the gym. We go a few times a week, and pound away on the treadmill or the exercise bike. The whole thing probably takes a couple of hours, by the time we have traveled there and back, had a shower, had a chat. But we feel virtuous. At the end of our first week we optimistically get back on the scales.

No change.

Ah well, obviously haven't been doing it for long enough, must keep going. So we continue going to the gym and at the end of a month discover that, despite all that time and effort, there has again been little change on the scales.

How is this possible? It is so unfair. We have been repeatedly told that if we do the exercise we will reap the reward, but we don't see any difference. It is at this point that our motivation slumps as we fail to see results and we realize we are going to have to put in hour after hour of slog for minimal gain. And then, like many before us who started out at the gym with good intentions, we give up.

If this happens to you then take some small consolation from the fact that you are not alone. As Dr. Stephen Boutcher of the School of Medical Sciences at the University of New South Wales has said, "Most exercise programs designed for weight loss have focused on steady state exercise of around 30 minutes at a moderate intensity on most days of the week. Disappointingly, these kinds of exercise programs have led to little or no loss."[9]

In the aerobic workout heyday of the 1980s and 90s it was universally accepted that we burn more calories from fat when working at lower intensities. Go steady, but go long, was the advice, and you will enter the "fat-burning zone." Jump on any older piece of cardio equipment and you'll see that the lower heart rate zone is still labeled "fat burning."

The truth is, however, that although you will burn some fat at low intensity, it won't be much and it won't make a significant dent in your paunch.

So why doesn't moderate-intensity exercise do what it is supposed to do, what we have been promised it will do? It should be straightforward. Do more exercise, burn more calories, lose more weight.

The problem is that, when it comes to humans, things are rarely straightforward.

Let's look at what happened in a study done at the University of Pittsburgh[10] where they followed nearly 200 overweight women for two years while they went through an intensive weight-loss program. The women were asked to make a big cut in their calorie intake—they had to consume less than 1,500 calories a day—and to significantly increase their exercise levels.

To make sure the women kept to the program they got lots of support. They were given treadmills to take home, they were encouraged to meet frequently, and they had regular phone calls urging them to keep going.

Initially, all went well. Six months after starting the program, more than half the women had lost at least 10% of their body weight and most were still doing regular exercise. Then, as often happens, things began to fall apart. Most of the women lapsed and started to regain the weight they had so painfully lost. Some did manage to keep going to the two-year mark, but to keep the weight off they were having to do significant amounts of exercise, nearly 70 minutes a day, five days a week.

So why is it so difficult to shed fat? Well, part of the problem is that fat is an incredibly energy-dense substance. A pound of fat contains more energy than a pound of dynamite. This means you have to do a lot of exercise to burn even a small amount of fat.

To find out just how much, I returned to Loughborough University where I was put through my paces by sports scientist Dr. Keith Tolfrey.

Keith asked me to wear a face mask attached to mobile monitoring equipment. The equipment, he told me, would measure the amount of oxygen I breathed in and the amount of carbon dioxide I breathed out. From that he could calculate the number of calories I burned while running.

Keith got me to run at a brisk pace around the track, while he cycled alongside shouting encouragement. I wasn't exactly going at Olympic pace, but I was going fast enough to feel relieved when, after ten minutes, Keith told me I could stop.

Then he and his colleagues gathered around the data-gathering machine and announced that I had consumed around 14 calories a minute, which meant that, having run a mile, I had burned through a grand total of . . . 140 calories. Not bad, I thought. But put it in perspective. A small bar of chocolate contains about 240 calories, while a large chocolate muffin comes in at an impressive 520 calories. So if you decide to have a muffin and a medium latte (150 calories) after your run, then you are topping yourself up with 670 calories.

And it gets worse, because the figures I just gave you are misleading. When you are judging the benefits of exercise you really should take into account that you would also be burning quite a lot of calories just by sitting down. The fact is that most of the calories we burn come from simply keeping our bodies going. So what you want to know is not the total calorie burn (TCB) but the net calorie burn (NCB), i.e., how many extra calories you burn by running rather than lying on the sofa. Funnily enough, you are rarely given this net figure. Perhaps because it might be discouraging.

To calculate your NCB from running a mile at a reasonable pace (doing six miles an hour, say, or walking at about three mph), use these formulas:

NCB from running a mile at moderate pace =
0.7 x your weight (in pounds)

NCB for walking a mile at around 3 mph =
0.4 x your weight (in pounds)

If you compare these figures with those you will find at popular websites, where they only give you the TCB, you will see they are rather lower.[11]

The one consoling fact about these formulas is that the heavier you are the more calories you will get through. When I did the run with Keith, I weighed 180 pounds, which meant that my NCB from running a mile was about 126 calories. Since then I have dropped to 160 pounds (through intermittent fasting), so I would now burn through 112 calories while covering the same distance.

My wife, who is 120 pounds, would get through just 78 calories running a mile, 48 calories walking a mile. Life is unfair.

Let's look at how far she would have to run or walk to burn through some common snacks or drinks.

	CALORIES	RUNNING	WALKING
Banana	90	1.1 miles	40 mins
Glass apple juice	120	1.5 miles	50 mins
Small glass wine/6 oz	126	1.6 miles	1 hour
Smoothie/8 oz	140–180	2 miles	1 hour 20 mins
Tall latte	180	2.2 miles	1 hour 30 mins
Large chocolate bar	240	3 miles	1 hour 40 mins
Large chocolate muffin	480	6 miles	3 hrs 20 mins

You can begin to see the difficulty of trying to lose weight through exercise alone.

There are roughly 3,500 calories in a pound of fat, which means that to shed a single pound of fat through exercise I would need to run at least an hour a day for six days. Or I could run a marathon. Either way, it is a lot of running.

Running, then, is not a great way of burning calories. What about other forms of exercise, like weight lifting? Dr. Jason Gill from Glasgow University has measured the calories you consume while doing this, and the results are even less impressive. "You burn more calories going for a gentle stroll than doing strenuous weight training," he told me.

"But surely weight training builds muscle and therefore increases your metabolic rate?" I protested.

"Yes, but not much," replied Jason. "If you trained hard for six months you would probably raise your daily metabolic rate by about 100 calories a day, which is the equivalent of a small glass of fruit juice."

This was discouraging. And there was more bad news. You might think, "Perhaps the reason I'm not losing weight despite doing lots of exercise is because I am turning fat into muscle and muscle is, of course, heavier than fat." Well, that could be true, but then again it probably isn't.

In a recent Australian study,[12] they took 45 overweight young women and randomly allocated them to different exercise regimes. One group was asked to cycle at moderate intensity, three times a week, 40 minutes at a time, for fifteen weeks. They were properly supervised to make sure they had done their exercise. At the end of the trial, just as they had at the beginning, they underwent a DXA scan to measure their body fat (for more on DXA scanning, see page 369). I would not have wanted to be the person who gave them the results, because after 30 hours of cycling they had, on average, put on a pound of fat.

How is this possible? Surely there must have been some mistake? Well, no, there is a painful but very obvious explanation. Studies show that when we begin to exercise most of us don't stick to our normal food intake. We often compensate by eating more. Sometimes a lot more. In fact, even the *thought* of exercise may encourage us to start eating.

In a study done at the University of Illinois, students were asked to evaluate the effectiveness of some lifestyle leaflets. The students were split into two groups. One group looked at leaflets encouraging them to do more exercise, the other group at leaflets which urged them to make friends. Afterwards they were asked to eat raisins, to rate their flavor. The students who had been shown the exercise leaflets ate a third more raisins than the other group.

Now this is hardly a real-world experiment, but there is plenty of evidence from the real world that we are prone to compensatory eating.

As Dr. Gill told me, "The initial effects of exercise are often to decrease appetite. The trouble is, we may decide to reward ourselves after a heavy session in the gym with a bar of chocolate or a full-fat cappuccino. There is evidence that we unconsciously eat to fill the energy gap, or compensate for increased activity by doing less when we are not exercising."

A Brief Explanation of Set Point Theory

The studies which suggest that your body will unconsciously try to sabotage your attempts to lose fat are supported by something called Set Point Theory. This theory is an attempt to explain why it is that so many people who try to lose weight through exercise, dieting, or some combination of the two, find it hard. The answer seems to be that your body will do all it can to keep your weight steady, at a particular set point.

Imagine you are overweight and decide to lose a few pounds. You go on a diet and increase the amount of exercise you do. Initially the weight drops off. Great. Then it slows. You have cut your calories and increased your activity but not much is happening. What's going on?

Well, as you lose weight your metabolic rate slows down, simply because you are carrying around less weight than you were before. But the amount your metabolic rate slows cannot be explained simply by weight loss. It seems that your body also becomes more efficient at storing and using calories.

The good news is that exercise will slow the rate at which your metabolic rate falls. The bad news is that it isn't as effective as we once hoped.

In a review study published in 2012, researchers asked plaintively, "Why do individuals not lose more weight from an exercise intervention?"[13]

The answer seems to be three-pronged: it's because even the experts underestimate how much exercise is needed to shift fat; because the volunteers in these studies compensate by eating more; and finally because exercise has less effect on keeping your metabolic rate revved up than previously believed.

This study was carried out at Penning Biomedical Research Center, where they have created an interesting and hopefully more accurate weight-loss predictor which you can use at: http://www.pbrc.edu/research-and-faculty/calculators/weight-loss-predictor/.

Based on this calculator, I can see that, if I start running for an hour a day, five days a week (without compensatory eating), then I will lose around three pounds in the first month. Not bad. But unless I increase the length or intensity of my run this rate of loss will soon slow. By the end of six months, my exercise regime will lead to about half that weight loss,

1.5 pounds a month. By the end of twelve months it's helping me lose just 0.1 pound a week. Effectively nothing.

So Should I Give Up Now?

Although this may all sound defeatist and gloomy there is good news as well.

For starters, there are benefits to exercise that go beyond weight. From a health point of view it is better to be fat and fit than lean and not fit.

In a study done at the Cooper Institute in Dallas, Texas,[14] researchers followed 22,000 men, aged between 30 and 83, for more than eight years. Before the study started the men had a full medical checkup, including a treadmill exercise test which tested their aerobic fitness. Over the eight years of follow-up, 427 of the men died, mainly from heart disease and cancer.

What they discovered in this study is that, when it comes to living longer, fitness is more important than fatness. The men who were overweight but fit were far less likely to die than the men who were normal weight but unfit. In fact, a fit overweight man was no more likely to die than a fit man of normal weight. (A similar study published in 2006 showed that the same is true of women.)

So if you want to live a long and healthy life it seems that being fit is more important than being slim.

Another thing about exercise is that although on its own it is not a great way of losing weight, when you combine it with a diet the combination is likely to be more effective than either done alone.

In a recently published study by Krista Varady and other researchers from the University of Illinois in Chicago,[15] 64 obese volunteers were randomly allocated to one of four groups: either ADF (alternate day fasting—i.e., eating a quarter of their normal calorie intake every other day) plus endurance exercise; ADF alone; endurance exercise alone; or a control group.

After twelve weeks, those doing ADF plus exercise had lost 6 kilograms (13.2 pounds), compared to 3 kilograms (6.5 pounds) for ADF alone and 1 kilogram (2.2 pounds) for exercise alone. Those doing the combined approach also saw the biggest improvements in cholesterol and fat loss. The researchers concluded that exercise plus dieting "produces superior changes in body weight, body composition, and lipid indicators of heart disease risk when compared to individual treatments."

In Summary

Exercise is clearly good for us—it's good for our mood, our general health, and our brains—but it is not a guaranteed way of losing weight. This is because:

★ Traditional low-intensity exercise is not a time-efficient way of burning fat

★ If you are going to lose weight and keep it off, exercise is not enough on its own—you also have to curb calories

★ After a bout of exercise, there is a tendency to indulge in a bout of compensatory eating. Try not to undo the good you have done through exercising by rewarding yourself with a high-calorie snack

★ We are also more likely to reduce the amount of activity we do after exercising. Look out for compensatory slacking . . .

Fret not! It is possible to get fitter and lose fat. Read on.

CHAPTER FIVE

What Is FastExercise?

HERE IS A PERSISTENT WIDESPREAD BELIEF IN THE fitness industry that the more time you spend exercising, the better. Only those who dedicate themselves to punishingly lengthy workouts can expect their body fat to plummet, their muscles to become exquisitely defined, to finally enter the kingdom of heavenly bodies. Tracey Anderson, trainer to Gwyneth Paltrow and Jennifer Lopez, famously said that she expects devotees of her method to spend 90 minutes a day on her regime. Madonna reportedly spends two hours a day with her trainer.

If that is how you wish to spend your time, good luck. If not, then you will be pleased to hear that the question occupying the minds of many of those at the forefront of exercise research is not so much "How can we get people to do more?" but "How can we get more for less?" HIT has caused a stir because studies done over the last decade have repeatedly shown that a few minutes of intense exercise a day can make a significant difference.

Yet the principles behind HIT are not new. Not even remotely new.

How the Hunter-Gatherers Did It

Each of us has a deep history. We are the product of thousands of generations of our species, a species that for most of its existence has lived precariously. Life for a caveman or woman was generally nasty, brutish, and short. To keep in shape they didn't "exercise"; they simply did a wide range of different activities that helped ensure that they survived and passed on their genes, eventually, to us. Our bodies and our genes were forged by the demands of the environment in which they lived. Perhaps by looking to the past we can learn how to stay in shape, and ensure that we have a future.

The problem, of course, is that our Pleistocene ancestors are long gone and it is impossible to say with great accuracy and simply by looking at their remains how they would have lived. The closest examples we have today of people who live much as our ancestors may have done are hunter-gatherers, people like the Hadza of northern Tanzania.

The Hadza live very near the Olduvai Gorge, part of the Great Rift Valley. Due to the large number of very ancient human fossils that have been found in the area it is sometimes known as the "Cradle of Mankind." In the surrounding land there is evidence of hominid occupation going back nearly two million years, including indications of *Homo erectus*, *Homo habilis*, and early *Homo sapiens*. Hunter-gatherers have been living in the area for at least 50,000 years and for much of that time the ancestors of the Hadza have been left untouched by "civilization." Until recently, the Hadza still hunted on foot using bows, axes, and digging sticks. They did not have cars or guns. They certainly did not have access to fast-food joints or gyms.

For some reason I had this idea that hunter-gatherers spend a lot of time traveling at a gentle jog, tracking game for days on end. In fact, when anthropologists started following the Hadza, they found that they don't do a lot unless they have to. In a study in which they asked the Hadza to wear GPS trackers and other sophisticated sensors, they found that, contrary to what you might expect, the number of calories they burn per pound of body weight is about the same as yours or mine.[1]

The reason they don't run about much is that they live on a relatively low-calorie diet. They need to conserve their energy. Instead of jogging, the men typically walk about seven miles (eleven kilometers) a day while hunting food. Women, who are less involved in hunting, cover more like four miles (six kilometers) a day. Both sexes do energy-sapping tasks like chopping wood and digging up tubers to eat, but they also do a lot of loafing around. Not surprisingly, they tend to be lean: a Hadza man in his midthirties typically has a body-fat percentage of 13%, a woman one of around 21%. This compares to the average in North America of 21% for men and 34% for women.

What is clear from studying hunter-gatherers is that they do a proper mix of different activities. They alternate low-intensity but fairly constant movement with short bursts of high-intensity activity (e.g., hunting, climbing trees, chopping wood). They also alternate periods of strenuous activity with days where they do relatively little.

As we'll show, there is compelling evidence that this hunter-gatherer approach is also good for our more coddled bodies. We need to be active, but not too active. We benefit from short bursts of intense activity and we need rest days to recover or we undo all the good work. As the authors of "Achieving Hunter-gatherer fitness in the 21st Century," a paper in the *American Journal of Medicine*,[2] point out,

> Hunter-gatherers would have likely alternated difficult days with less demanding days when possible. The same pattern of alternating a strenuous workout one day with an easy one the next day produces higher levels of fitness with lower rates of injury. . . . The natural cross-training that was a mandatory aspect of life as a hunter-gatherer improves performance across many athletic disciplines.

In fact, the authors are so convinced that a hunter-gatherer lifestyle is beneficial that they put together what they call "The characteristics of a Hunter-gatherer Fitness Program." According to this, if you want to exercise like a hunter-gatherer, you should:

1. Do a lot of light background activity such as walking.

2. Have hard days followed by easy days. You need rest, relaxation, and sleep.

3. Include interval training: short intermittent bursts of moderate- to high-intensity exercise interspersed with rest and recovery, 2–3 times a week.

4. Make sure you do regular sessions of strength- and flexibility-building. Hunter-gatherers have to chop wood, climb trees, or carry a child around.

5. Ideally do all exercise outdoors, where you get exposed to sunlight, which gives your skin a chance to generate vitamin D. Although it is called a vitamin, "vitamin" D is actually a hormone, with a far wider range of activity than people had previously imagined. Many of us, particularly those who live in the northern hemisphere, are chronically short of vitamin D.

6. Try to do as much exercise as possible in a social setting. We are intensely social creatures and doing exercise together is a good way of ensuring that we do it at all.

FastExercise is based on the hunter-gatherer approach. In Chapter 6, Peta offers a range of workouts that use different forms of HIT, many of which can be done outdoors; and in Chapter 8, I describe ways in which you can build more activity into your life. But before we come to that, let's look at the story behind the discovery of HIT.

A Short History of HIT

One of the first people to use high-intensity interval training and to study it scientifically was an early twentieth-century German coach named Woldemar Gerschler. He was, by all accounts, an extremely demanding man, but a man who was passionately interested in the science of exercise.

The athletes who trained with him were typically asked to sprint 100, 200, sometimes 400 meters at a pace that would get their hearts up to 180 beats per minute. They would then wait till their heart rate dropped to 120, before doing it again. Gerschler had realized that it was the combination of intensity and recovery that was critical.

Gerschler showed that in less than three weeks he could increase an athlete's heart volume by 20% and make significant improvements in their race times. His students began to put together some truly remarkable performances.

In 1939 Rudolf Harbig, a runner coached by Gerschler, broke the world 800-meter record by a massive 1.6 seconds. The following month he broke the world 400-meter record as well. His 800-meter record lasted sixteen years, until in 1955 Roger Moens, an athlete who was also coached by Gerschler, ran it in 1:45.7.

Meanwhile, in 1950s Britain, a young medical student, Roger Bannister, was determined to become the first person in the world to run a sub-four-minute mile. The trouble was, as a busy student he didn't have lots of spare time for training. So he would go down to the track and do interval sprints. These consisted of running flat-out for about 1 minute, during which time he would cover a quarter of a mile (440 yards, about 400 meters). Then he would jog for 2–3 minutes before doing another one-minute sprint. He would repeat this cycle 10 times, then head back to work. Since he rarely bothered with much in the way of warm-ups or cooldowns, the whole thing normally took less than 35 minutes.

In May 1954, Roger Bannister took part in a race at the Iffley Road track in Oxford, which he duly won. The announcer, Norris McWhirter (who went on to coedit the *Guinness Book of Records*), clearly enjoyed his share of what would turn out to be a great sporting moment. Slowly, ponderously, he spelled out the results: "Ladies and gentlemen, here is the result of event nine, the one mile: first, No. 41, R. G. Bannister, Amateur Athletic Association and formerly of Exeter and Merton Colleges, Oxford, with a time which is a new meeting and track record, and which—subject to ratification—will be a new English Native, British National, All-Comers, European, British Empire and World Record. The time was three . . ."

There was a huge roar which drowned out the rest of the message as the crowd realized that the "three . . ." must mean they had just watched the first person to run the mile in less than four minutes.

What I find particularly interesting about this story is that Roger Bannister's regime—10 sets of one-minute sprints, split by a couple of minutes of recovery—is now widely used by HIT enthusiasts, and not, as we'll see, just by serious runners but by the overweight, the unfit, and those with previous histories of cardiac problems. It is also the way that Peta likes to train.

Other incredibly successful middle-distance athletes have used different HIT regimes. Sebastian Coe, who once held world records in the 800 meters, the mile, and the 1,500 meters at the same time, did fast sprints with short recoveries, but in his case it was more likely to be 20-second sprints with 30 seconds of recovery. That is my preferred regime, too—though I do it on a bicycle and only manage to do it about three times before collapsing.

HIT and Elite Athletes

When Coe was breaking world records in the 1970s, HIT was still relatively little used and seen mainly as a way of increasing speed, not endurance. These days there is un-likely to be any athlete who has reached the top in any sport without having made this sort of exercise at least part of their workload.

It's pretty obvious that athletes who engage in sports that require stop-start bursts of speed—tennis, football, squash, hockey, and martial arts—will benefit from HIT. In many ways the HIT approach simulates what they will experience in competition—including the buildup of waste products in tired limbs and the need to override those almost crippling effects to be able to sprint again. And again. And again.

Cyclists, sprinters, and swimmers who compete in shorter distance races have to learn to push themselves to the limit in one training session, but ensure that their bodies have recovered for the next. For all of these, HIT-type training several times a week is a tried and tested solution.

What is more surprising is how important HIT is for endurance athletes. For elite long-distance cyclists, marathon runners, triathletes, race-walkers, and open-water swimmers, variations of HIT increasingly form a big part of their training program. HIT—by putting the body under stress and increasing mitochondrial activity (which we'll come to in depth later)—adds to explosive power.

In short, HIT allows athletes to run, swim, and cycle faster for longer. It prepares them for the discomfort that comes from extremes of effort and primes their bodies to deal with the worst that high-level competition can throw at them. And to finish on top.

What About the Rest of Us?

The trouble with trying to extrapolate from studies with trained athletes is that these people are, almost by definition, unlike the rest of us. What can HIT do for us lesser mortals? Over the last two decades lots of researchers around the world have studied the effects of HIT in different populations, but the man who has done more than most is Martin Gibala, Professor of Exercise Science at McMaster University in Canada.

Back in 2005, he and his colleagues published a study which had a huge impact on the exercise world.[3]

They asked eight reasonably active young volunteers to do six sessions of what they called SIT—sprint interval training. Training consisted of between four and seven sessions, carried out over two weeks, with 1–2 days rest in between each session.

SIT is a real misnomer. It sounds easy. It is not. You get on a special bike and, after a brief warm-up, you have to cycle flat-out for 30 seconds against resistance. You then have a breather that lasts about four minutes, which you spend gently pedaling, then you do another 30-second sprint. Gradually you build it up. When the brave volunteers did it back in the mid-1990s, they were doing this up to seven times in each session.

It is difficult to imagine how tough this really is. The first 30-second burst is OK. You think to yourself, "That was manageable." The next 30-second burst is hard. You really welcome the four-minute break. The third time, you cannot believe how slowly the seconds go past. The pedals slow; you have to focus to try and keep up speed. By the time you get to number seven (if you ever get to number seven) you are truly exhausted and need to lie down on the sofa for a while.

SIT is tiring, but the time commitment is very low. In total the SIT volunteers did only fifteen minutes of hard exercise across the two weeks and those fifteen minutes made some impressive differences.

The volunteers' "cycle endurance capacity," their ability to push themselves hard on a bike, doubled. Whereas previously they had managed to cycle hard for 26 minutes, now they could do it for 51 minutes. Something remarkable had gone on inside their bodies.

But what?

Martin Gibala did another study.[4]

This time he decided (or his volunteers told him) that doing seven sets of 30 seconds per session was too much for a normal human to endure. So he generously cut it down to a maximum of six.

He enlisted 16 young men (these studies are often but not exclusively done with men, probably because men are more likely to be found hanging around science labs) and randomly divided them into two groups.

Eight were asked to do six sessions of cycling at reasonable intensity for 1½ to 2 hours at a time.

The other group also did six sessions, but with short bursts of flat-out cycling. In each session they did 2–3 minutes of intense exercise, which along with the recovery periods meant each session lasted about twenty minutes.

At the end of training the steady-cycling volunteers had spent more than ten hours on their bikes, while the SIT lot had done just over two hours.

When researchers did the the follow-up tests (including muscle biopsies, which I can tell you from personal experience are not pleasant), they found that both groups had improved on a whole range of measures by much the same amount. The difference was that it had taken the SIT group a fifth of the time.

Making It Easier: The Bannister Method

By now, Martin and his colleagues realized that doing 30-second bursts of flat-out cycling would be a challenge for people who were not already pretty fit. SIT, as Martin explained, "is extremely demanding and it may not be safe, tolerable or appealing for some individuals."

So they broke it down further, into a protocol that they believed could be safely done by people who are unfit, overweight, or have a previous history of heart disease, stroke, or diabetes.[5]

The new protocol consisted of doing ten bursts of one-minute sprints, separated by one minute of recovery. This sort of protocol is somewhat similar to the one I described earlier, used by Roger Bannister when he was training to break the four-minute mile.

The main difference is that during those one-minute sprints you are not going flat-out. Instead you should be aiming to cycle hard enough to raise your pulse to about 80–90% of your maximal heart rate (to find out how to calculate this, see the "Ways to Measure the Impact of Exercise" section at the back). From my experience it is tough but bearable. It is also delightfully brief.

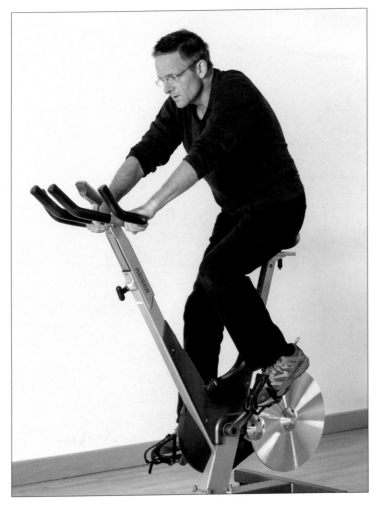

Indoor cycling is a good way of getting HIT because a modern indoor bike lets you add resistance, changing the intensity of the ride.

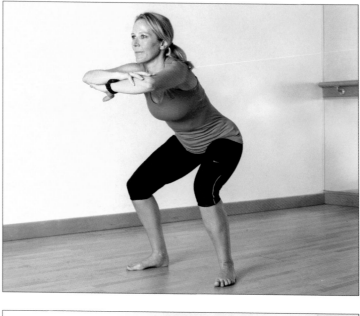

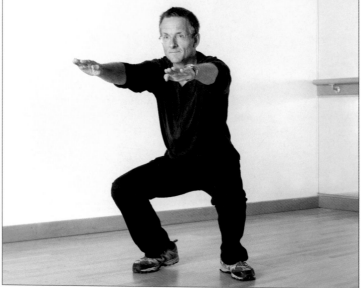

When squatting, bend from the hips, keeping the weight in your heels. Make sure your back is straight. Keep bending until the legs are at a 90-degree angle—imagine you are preparing to sit in a chair.

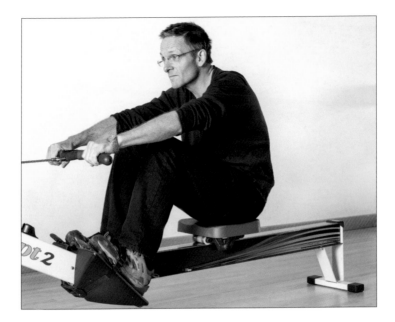

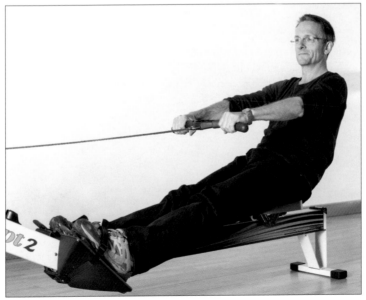

With rowing, good technique is crucial. Start each stroke by pushing with the legs, not pulling with the arms, and keep your wrists in line with the handle so that the cable is parallel to the floor.

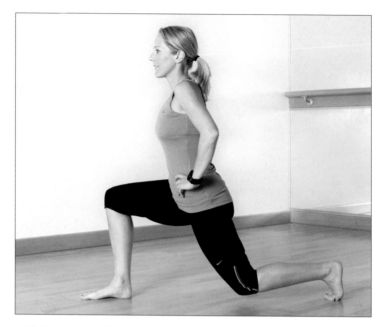

With lunges, step forward with one leg, bending both knees to 90 degrees and keeping your upper body straight.

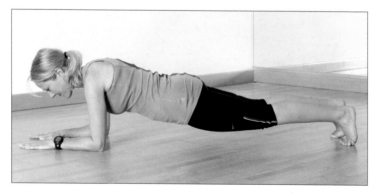

When doing the plank, make sure your midsection doesn't rise or drop. Squeeze your buttocks and hold the position for as long as possible. Remember, it should never cause pain in the lower back.

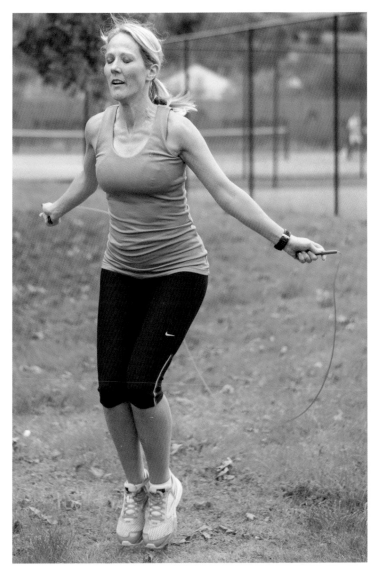

For jumping rope, knees and ankles should be flexed but your torso kept straight when jumping. Arms should be at your side with the rope turning from the wrists and forearms.

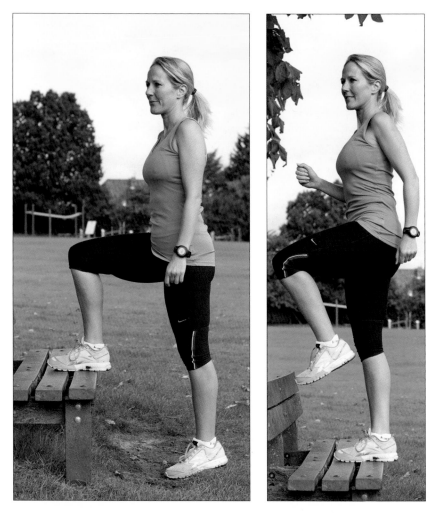

Chair step-ups should be performed with care but at a brisk pace. Place one foot on the "step" making sure your full foot is in contact with the surface. Push your body weight up, driving your weight through the heel and breathing out as you do this.

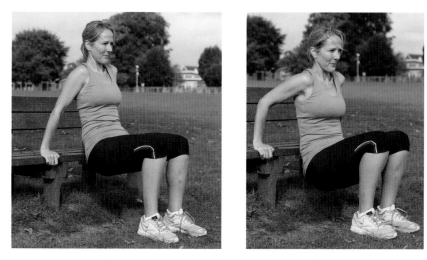

For tricep dips, place your palms on the seat behind you, bending your knees at right angles, hips straight. Bend your elbows to 90 degrees to lower your body (so that your bottom descends halfway to the floor).

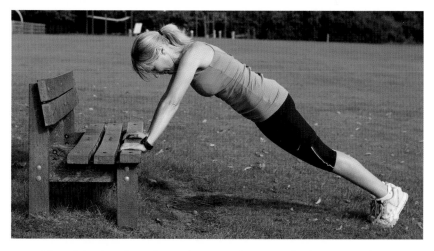

When doing bench push-ups, be sure to keep your body in a straight line, so that your weight is supported on the balls of your feet and by the elbows. Don't allow your back to arch or your hips to drop.

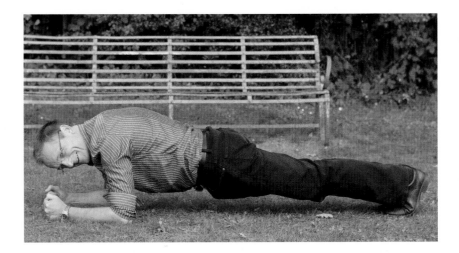

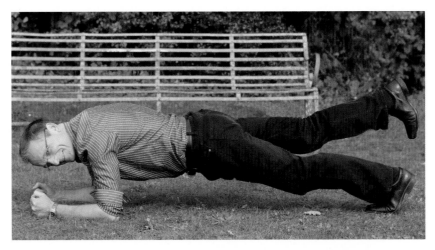

For a plank with leg raise, your elbows should be bent at a 90-degree angle. Keep your back straight with your hips raised off the floor. Squeeze the torso tight, slowly lifting one foot approximately 6–8 inches off the ground and hold the position for a few seconds.

So How Does HIT Work, and What Difference Does It Make?

There have been dozens of studies of different forms of HIT. Most have been quite short (a couple of weeks); some have lasted a few months. And so far only a few hundred people have been intensively studied (though the results of some big studies are expected soon).

Nonetheless, what the studies done so far consistently show is that:

★ HIT will get you aerobically fitter faster than standard exercise

★ HIT will improve insulin sensitivity faster than standard exercise

★ If you want to build muscle tone and lose some fat HIT is the most time-efficient way to achieve this

Let's look at the science behind HIT, and how it actually works.

Mitochondria or Power Cells

One of the reasons why doing HIT produces big changes in a short time is because of the effect that high-intensity exercise has on your mitochondria.

Mitochondria are the body's main power plants. Their job is to convert raw materials like oxygen and glucose into little packages of energy called ATP (adenosine triphosphate). The ATP is then used to power your body.

But mitochondria are much more than that. As Nick Lane puts it in his 2005 book, *Power, Sex, Suicide,* they are the "clandestine rulers of the world." Despite the fact that they are so small (a billion could fit in a grain of sand), they are the great turbochargers of life, responsible for the extraordinary range of creatures that live on earth today, including us.

There are mitochondria in every cell of your body, ranging from a few to many thousands. They are unlike anything else in your body because they have their own DNA, which is closer to that of bacteria than to that of human beings. They are interlopers, aliens, yet they are essential to our existence. Their long and fascinating history is, I think, worth a brief digression.

If we could travel back a few billion years, we would discover a profoundly different Earth. The days would be shorter, the atmosphere almost devoid of oxygen, and the continents would be completely unrecognizable. There would be no trees, no plants, no animals. In fact, the only forms of life you would encounter would be tiny single-celled microbes. These microbes got their energy through fermentation, breaking down complex compounds, and thrived in the anaerobic (oxygen-free) atmosphere of ancient Earth.

Then, around two billion years ago, a new creature appeared. It was a microbe with a difference, one that would change everything. This new microbe had acquired the ability to use sunlight as a source of power. It was a microbe that could photosynthesize.

Unfortunately for the other microscopic creatures that were living on our planet, generating energy through photosynthesis led to the release of an extremely toxic gas as a by-product. Over tens of millions of years the levels of this poisonous gas increased from virtually nothing to almost 21% of the entire atmosphere. It was the worst outbreak of pollution that this world has ever known and resulted in the death of countless life forms.

The by-product of photosynthesis was, of course, oxygen—and the effects of its increased levels in the atmosphere were so dramatic that the period has been labeled the Oxygen Catastrophe or Oxygen Crisis.

What the new supermicrobes that "invented" photosynthesis had done was use energy from sunlight to split water (H_2O) into oxygen and hydrogen. They mixed hydrogen with carbon to make simple sugars (i.e., food) and the oxygen was just released into the atmosphere.

While we think of oxygen as life-giving, it's actually extremely toxic. It reacts hungrily with proteins and enzymes, stopping them from working; it causes metal to rust. If levels rose much above where they are at present, trees would burst spontaneously into flames.

The reason why oxygen levels didn't simply go on rising is that eventually a new breed of microbes evolved an even smarter chemical trick—they learned how to convert oxygen, the great poison, into energy.

The microbes that did this were an early ancestor of the tiny mitochondria that now live happily inside our cells. We have acquired, through them, the ability to use oxygen as a fuel. We can also, thanks to even earlier microscopic ancestors, produce energy anaerobically (without oxygen), though this is a far less efficient process. So when people talk about doing aerobic exercise they are really talking about doing a form of exercise that depends primarily on getting mitochondria to produce power.

I've gone on at length about mitochondria because they are important for understanding how HIT works. Since mitochondria produce power, then, broadly speaking, you want more of them. One way to produce more is to do exercise. In fact, a good measure of how effective an exercise regime is going to be is whether it results in greater mitochondrial density.

And that's where HIT seems to score particularly well. Doing HIT leads to the production of greater numbers of more active mitochondria than doing standard exercise will. This is true not just in skeletal muscle (i.e., the muscles that make you move) but also heart muscle (the muscle that keeps you alive).

HIT makes heart muscle bigger and more efficient. After doing HIT your heart muscle needs less oxygen to do the same amount of work. In short, doing HIT leads to a bigger, stronger heart.

This is important because one of the main fears about doing HIT is that it could trigger a heart attack or stroke. In fact, there is convincing evidence that doing HIT will *reduce* the risk of this happening and will also help you recover faster after a heart attack. It's a promising but still controversial area of research which I will return to later.

FastExercise and Fat

The other good thing about mitochondria is that they burn fat. So if HIT makes more mitochondria it should lead to more fat burning. But what's the evidence? Well, let's return once more to the Australian study—in which 45 women were randomly allocated to either 3 x 40 minutes of moderate-intensity cycling a week (see page 240) or three 20-minute sessions of higher-intensity intermittent cycling.[6]

The women who had been allocated to the high-intensity group were asked to alternate eight seconds of sprint cycling with twelve seconds of gentle cycling. They started doing this for five minutes, building up to twenty minutes per session.

At the end of fifteen weeks, both groups had got fitter, as measured by improvements in their aerobic fitness, or VO2 max, but only the high-intensity group had lost any weight. They lost an average of 2.5 kilograms (5.5 pounds)—but within this average there was huge variability. Some of the women lost up to 8 kilograms (17.6 pounds), a few lost very little. The ones who lost very little were the ones who were lean to begin with. The fatter the women were at the start of the study, the more fat they had lost by the end.

However, the women who did normal moderate-intensity

cycling, despite spending twice as long on their bikes, managed to put on weight and became slightly fatter.

The particularly good news from this study was that the women doing the HIT lost fat not only from their thighs, which you might expect, but also from their stomachs. The reduction in abdominal fat was accompanied by a decrease in fasting insulin, down by 31%.

If you were wondering if the same is true of men, the research team did a similar study using young overweight males. They recruited 46 inactive, overweight young men (aged around 25) and got them to do three 20-minute sessions a week on an exercise bike. Like the women, after a brief warm-up, they had to sprint for eight seconds, then cycle gently for twelve seconds. The idea was to try and keep their heart rate racing along at around 80–90% of maximum while sprinting. In men this age that would mean pushing the heart rate up to around 160 beats per minute.[7]

After 6 weeks there was not much change in body fat, which must have been discouraging. Then, however, the changes really began to kick in. By the end of twelve weeks the young men's aerobic power had increased by 15% and on average they had lost 2 kilograms (4.4 pounds) of fat. Encouragingly, they had lost a lot of that fat from the gut (visceral fat was down by 17%) and they had put on muscle.

Compared to the Australian women who had done a similar regime they put on far more muscle, particularly in the thighs. They had also managed to do it in less time, as this trial ran for twelve weeks rather than fifteen.

In another study from the University of Ontario,[8] ten

men and ten women were randomly allocated to do HIT or to do lengthy runs three times a week for six weeks. Unlike the Australian volunteers, who did eight seconds of intense cycling followed by twelve seconds' dawdling, this lot were asked to perform 4–6 bursts of 30-second sprints with a recovery period of four minutes between each burst.

The control group was asked to run on a treadmill for 60 minutes at a steady pace that raised their heart rate to around 65% of maximum.

At the end of the trial, the steady runners had lost some body fat, but the HIT exercisers had shed more than twice as much, an impressive 12.4% of their fat mass. And they had done it in a fraction of the time.

How Does Turning Up the HIT Burn Fat?

★ When you push the intensity of a workout, you build more metabolically active muscle, and because muscle is efficient at burning fat your total calorie expenditure soars. This happens mainly because HIT makes the muscle cells produce new and more active mitochondria, power plants that transfer fat into energy and heat. The mitochondria not only burn fat when you are exercising but go on doing so for some time afterwards as your muscles recover.

★ The metabolic stress caused by HIT also leads to a huge increase in the production of catecholamines— hormones like adrenaline and noradrenaline—

that lead to much greater fat burning. As Dr. John Babraj and Dr. Ross Lorimer point out in their book, *The High Intensity Workout*: "Adrenaline and noradrenaline are elevated by as much as 1450% following a high-intensity training session. The size of the response is much bigger than is seen with steady exercise such as jogging or cycling."

★ So why does HIT lead to fat loss in your gut? Well, one reason is that there are more catecholamine receptors in abdominal fat than in subcutaneous fat, so when you get a surge of catecholamines following a vigorous burst of HIT, they target abdominal fat, increasing the release of fat from visceral fat stores.

★ Catecholamines also activate brown fat (see box below), which burns rather than stores energy.

★ High-intensity training also seems to suppress appetite in ways that low-intensity exercise does not.

A Note on Brown Fat

More than 30 years ago I watched a science documentary about something called "brown fat." Unlike normal fat, brown fat contains a lot more mitochondria, which is what makes it brown. Brown fat is most commonly found in newborn babies and in hibernating mammals. It is there, primarily, to generate heat. Unlike the more familiar yellowish-white body fat that stores excess calories, brown fat does the opposite. It burns calories. When "switched on," brown fat produces around 300 times more heat than any other organ in the body.

Back in the 1980s it was thought that activating brown fat would be one way to solve the obesity problem. But things didn't work out so well. Though it had been known for some time that babies have deposits of brown fat around their shoulder blades to help them maintain their body temperature (babies are not very good at shivering), scientists couldn't find brown fat in adults. So they decided brown fat must disappear in infancy once it is no longer really needed. Interest in brown fat dwindled. Recently, thanks to better technology, it has returned.

In the last decade, researchers carrying out PET-CT scans have found traces of brown fat in adults, particularly on the upper back, the side of the neck, in the dip between the collarbone and the shoulder, and along the spine. Not a lot, but enough to encourage further investigation.

It turns out women have proportionately more brown fat than men and it is more readily detectable in lean people than in the obese, although researchers are still not sure why. What's now accepted is that brown fat persists into adulthood and that there are a couple of ways of activating it. What we don't yet know is how big or significant this effect is likely to be.

High-intensity exercise certainly leads to a flood of hormones like noradrenaline, known to activate brown fat. Exposure to cold will also encourage your brown fat to burn through a few more calories. Using thermal-imaging techniques, researchers at the University of Nottingham's Queen's Medical Centre have shown that plunging your hands into a bucket of cold water can trigger brown fat into calorie-burning action. Likewise, exercise in the cold can boost the fat-burning effect, one reason to turn the thermostat down and go out for a stroll on a cold winter's night.

HIT and Appetite

Any form of exercise will lead to some fat burning; but, as we've seen already, unless you also curb your calories it will not lead to weight loss. So what effect does HIT have on appetite?

In a trial conducted in 2011,[9] 15 obese adolescent French boys were asked to spend a few days in a metabolic chamber, a room equipped with bed, TV, toilet, exercise bike, and not much else. The scientists were able to keep a really close eye on exactly what the boys were up to and what was happening to their metabolisms.

At 8 a.m. the boys went into the chamber and ate a carefully measured breakfast. A couple of hours later they were asked to do a session of either high- or low-intensity cycling (they had to alternate: one day "high" followed by one day "low," or vice versa). Whether they were doing high- or low-intensity cycling, the boys had to keep going until they had burned off exactly 330 calories.

Thirty minutes after exercising they were offered a buffet lunch, which they tucked into. Buffets are a popular research tool because people just help themselves and are not influenced by the amount of food they are offered.

After lunch the boys were encouraged to be idle for the rest of the day before eating whatever they fancied from a buffet dinner. Then they went to bed.

The boys filled in diaries which showed they didn't notice any difference in their appetite after doing the different levels of exercise nor did they consciously change how much they ate.

Nonetheless, on the days they did high-intensity cycling they ate significantly less at the two buffet meals than when they did low-intensity exercise.

At lunch, for example, the boys ate 10% less after high-intensity exercise than after a less intense session. Even more striking was the buffet dinner, where they ate 20% less than they had on less active days.

The finding from this study is consistent with others which have found that the effects of high-intensity exercise on appetite peak around seven hours after a single bout.

So HIT seems to curb appetite, at least for a while. Unfortunately, the effect of doing HIT does wear off. The following morning (twenty hours after exercising) the boys ate just as much breakfast whether they had exercised the previous day or not.

The researchers of this particular study are not entirely sure why high-intensity exercise suppresses appetite. They think it might be because of the effect it has on hormones that regulate appetite, such as PYY (see box on pages 271–273), glucagon-like peptide 1, or leptin. They also acknowledge that "questions still remain as to whether the anorexic effect of HIE [anorexic, as in loss of appetite] can be maintained during prolonged training."

So, does HIT really lead to long-term appetite suppression? The short answer is that we simply don't know; there have not been sufficient long-term trials yet. But the results from the two Australian studies I mentioned earlier, which ran for three months and showed significant fat loss from HIT, suggest it might.

Interestingly, another group of Australian researchers showed that the more intense the exercise, the longer it suppresses appetite. They took overweight young men in their twenties and early thirties and got them to ride on a stationary bike for 30 minutes, with one minute of high-intensity cycling followed by four minutes of gentle pedaling.

This time, however, they threw in a fourth day when the men had to put themselves through a much tougher version of HIT, cycling for fifteen seconds of maximal effort followed by just one minute of rest, done for half an hour. They called this very high-intensity or VHI.

After each session the men were given a liquid meal containing 300 calories. Then, an hour later, they were offered porridge and told to eat as much as they wanted until they were "comfortably full."

Results published in the *International Journal of Obesity*[10] showed that the young men ate fewer calories after the high-intensity (621 calories) and very high-intensity (594 calories) workouts than they did after a bout of moderate exercise (710 calories).

Even more encouragingly, the men reported eating fewer calories on the day *following* the highest-intensity workout (2,000 calories) than they did after the moderate session (2,300 calories) or after resting (2,600 calories). As I mentioned above, this suggests that if you do extremely high-intensity exercise the effects of appetite suppression last far longer, well into the following day.

They also found some significant differences in the blood of their volunteers. There were, for example, lower levels of ghrelin, a hunger-promoting hormone, after doing intense exercise than after the gentler versions and there were also higher levels of lactate, which reduces appetite.

Another positive finding was that, although doing HIT was an effort, the men said they had enjoyed the more grueling version of the exercises.

HIT and Hunger Hormones

One of the hottest areas of clinical research, when it comes to weight loss, is the study of hormones produced by your body that control appetite—sometimes referred to as hunger hormones. Ghrelin, for example—a hormone produced by cells in the stomach—seems to increase appetite, while the hormones leptin and peptide YY (also known as PYY) reduce it.

Lots of studies have shown that ghrelin (I remember it as the GREEDY hormone) levels go up before a meal and fall after you have eaten. When you lose weight, average ghrelin levels also tend to rise, encouraging you to eat more and put the weight back on, which is annoying. A bout of insomnia will also make ghrelin levels rise, one reason why chronic sleep shortage can lead to weight gain.

We know that intense exercise will lower your ghrelin levels. What we don't know is how long the effect lasts and whether, in time, your body adjusts.

Leptin has also been intensely studied. Unlike ghrelin, it reduces your appetite. Think of it as the LEAN hormone. Leptin is made in fat tissue and controls your appetite by acting on the hypothalamus, a portion of the brain, suppressing hunger signals. There was, at one time, a widespread hope that a simple injection of leptin would suppress appetite in obese patients and, hey presto, the fat would just melt away. Unfortunately, it has not turned out to be anything like that easy.

Researchers soon discovered that most obese humans are not deficient in leptin. Far from it. They often have extremely high circulating levels of leptin. It seems that once you become obese, your cells become insensitive to leptin, and so your body responds by producing increasing amounts of it. In this respect it is rather like the levels of insulin, which also tend to rise as people become obese and their bodies become increasingly insensitive to its effects.

In the Australian study on young, overweight women outlined in the previous chapter (see page 240), the researchers found that insulin and leptin levels both fell significantly as the women doing HIT lost weight and got fitter. There were no changes in the women doing steady, low-intensity exercise.

My HIT Journey

When I first heard about HIT I was curious but skeptical. I liked the idea of getting fit in a short period of time and I particularly liked the idea of improving my insulin sensitivity as my father had died of diabetes-related illnesses and I could see the same thing happening to me.

The form of HIT I decided to start with was three bouts of twenty seconds, three times a week for four weeks. My mentor, Professor Jamie Timmons of Loughborough University, assured me that this sort of regime typically results in improvements in insulin sensitivity of around 25% and increased VO2 max (see page 231) of around 10%. He also warned me that these were average figures, which meant that I might do better than this, or considerably worse.

Before Jamie put me on his short, sharp regime, he measured my glucose tolerance and my VO2 max. I went into the lab, having fasted overnight, and on an empty stomach drank a glass of something with the equivalent of fifteen teaspoons of sugar in it. It was disgusting. Then I had to lie down while they took blood samples every ten minutes for the next two hours.

Jamie came to me with the results. I could tell from his face that the news was not particularly good.

"Your results are not perfect," Jamie said. "Your blood glucose went up after drinking all that sugar and then it slowly drifted down, just below the level we would call impaired glucose tolerance. So you're just within the healthy range. But only just."

With that unsettling discovery rattling around inside my head, I got on an exercise bike so they could measure my VO2 max. For the next twenty minutes I pushed myself to my absolute limit, hoping that these results would be a little more encouraging. My VO2 max score, 37 mL/(kg. min)—milliliters of oxygen per kilogram of body weight per minute—was not outstanding but it was at least acceptable. I would have preferred "world class" but had to settle for "good for your age."

With those results under my belt, I went away to do HIT on a special exercise bike that Jamie lent me. For the next four weeks I sprinted my little heart out on that exercise bike for exactly one minute a day, three days a week. I enjoyed the fact that it was so brief and the challenge of really pushing myself, but I discovered that even twenty seconds at full speed against resistance can make your thighs burn.

Just to see if it could be done, I sometimes tried doing the sprints in a suit and tie. The answer is yes: because the actual exercise was so brief, I never got uncomfortably hot, let alone sweaty.

After four weeks I went back to the lab to be retested. I drank the nauseatingly sweet drink and pushed myself as hard as possible on the bike.

Then it was time for my results. There was good news, and bad news. The good news was that my insulin sensitivity had improved by a remarkable 25%, exactly in line with Jamie's predictions. I was elated, and wondered why this had happened.

Jamie is not exactly sure, but he thinks that one way HIT works is that it disrupts glycogen stores—glucose that's stored in muscles. "The key thing about this form of exercise is that because it is vigorous it really breaks down the glycogen stores in the muscle and that's a signal from the muscle to the bloodstream saying I need to take up more glucose. Unlike walking or jogging where you may only be activating 20–30% of your muscle tissue, here you're activating 70–80%, so you're really creating a much bigger sink to soak up the glucose that follows a meal."

That was the good news. My increased insulin sensitivity suggested that I had, for the time being, reduced the risk that I would become a full-fledged diabetic.

Me and My Glucose

Unless you keep doing it the benefits of any exercise regime will wear off. To find out how quickly, in early 2012 I stopped doing HIT. Within a couple of months my blood glucose levels had returned to borderline diabetic.

At that point, rather than resume HIT, I decided to make myself the subject of another documentary in which I tested IF, intermittent fasting. As I describe in my book *The FastDiet*, on this regime I lost 20 pounds, most of it fat, and my blood glucose once more returned to normal.

These days I maintain my weight and improved glucose control through a combination of intermittent fasting and FastExercise.

The bad news was that, although I was able to push myself longer and harder on the exercise bike than I had on my previous visit and felt good about it, my aerobic fitness had not significantly improved. Despite sticking to the protocol, my heart and lungs were apparently in no better shape than they had been before I began doing HIT.

Although Jamie had warned me this might happen, it was still a nasty shock.

So why didn't HIT improve my aerobic fitness in the way that it had improved my insulin sensitivity? Why does it work better for some people than for others? The answer, as so often seems to be the case, lies in the genes.

The Genetics of Exercise

As I wrote at the beginning of this chapter, one of the most widely accepted beliefs about exercise is that the more you do the fitter you become. Like the link between exercise and weight loss, it seems so self-evidently true, so in line with common sense, that it is madness to suggest otherwise. Perhaps you will never become an Olympic athlete or run the mile in less than ten minutes, but if you train regularly then surely you must be making your heart and lungs stronger, adding years to your life. Sadly, life is not that fair.

"What we've known for quite some time now," Jamie said, "is that there's a huge variation in how people respond to an exercise regime and there's actually no guarantee that following any particular recipe will produce favorable results."

There have, in fact, been a number of studies showing that the extent to which people respond to exercise varies wildly from person to person. In a recent study from Finland,[11] 175 untrained, middle-aged volunteers (89 men and 86 women) were asked to do a 21-week training course. The volunteers either did strength training (lifting weights) twice a week, endurance training twice a week, or a workout which combined strength and endurance training four times a week.

The volunteers were carefully supervised to make sure they were actually doing the training and extensively tested before and after, measuring things like VO2 max and muscular strength.

The results were, to say the least, mixed. Some people's aerobic fitness improved by an impressive 42%, while others actually became less fit—their VO2 max dropped by 8%.

There was an even greater spread when it came to the strength exercises, with some people increasing their power output by 87% and others performing 12% worse at the end than they had at the beginning.

If this was the only study you might suspect that these were freakish results or that some of the volunteers were slacking. But there have been quite a number of studies that have come up with similar findings. The phenomenon has not been much commented on before because scientists tend to lump all data together and look for "average" results. Anomalies get ignored, treated as outliers.

The implication of this and other studies, however, is that there is a huge range in people's responses to exercise—from superresponders at one end of the spectrum, those who will get a lot of benefit from doing regular exercise, to nonresponders at the other, who are likely to get little.

So How Do You Know Whether You Are a So-Called Superresponder or a Nonresponder?

The most reliable way to get an answer to this question would be to do what the volunteers did in the Finnish trial: get yourself measured and then put yourself through 21 weeks of hard training. That way you would find out which end of the spectrum you belong to. The other option might be to have a blood test.

When Jamie and his collaborators investigated the reasons for the variations in people's response to exercise, they discovered that when it comes to aerobic fitness much of the difference can be traced to the genetic code contained within just 11 genes. On the basis of this finding they developed a genetic test that they claim can accurately predict how well an individual will respond to exercise.

Before starting my HIT program Jamie took a sample of my blood and sent it off to be DNA-tested. He didn't tell me the results until I'd done my four weeks of HIT.

After I had come back, been retested, and expressed disappointment that my aerobic fitness had not improved in line with my expectations (from the studies, I was hoping for at least a 10% improvement), Jamie brought out the results of my genetic test. They were not good. Or rather, from his perspective, they were very good.

Of the more than 700 people they had tested at that time, my results were among the lowest. I had the fewest "positive" versions of the genes that seem to promote improvements in VO2 max. As soon as he saw these results Jamie had been convinced that I would be a nonresponder when it came to improving aerobic fitness. He was right.

As a human being I'm sure he would have been delighted to give me better news, but as a scientist he was quietly pleased at the accuracy of his predictions.

I was naturally profoundly disappointed, but also not

wholly surprised. I think, in my bones, I have always known that exercise doesn't do for me what it seems to do for a lot of other people.

That said, I don't believe that genes are destiny, so I take these sorts of tests with a pinch of salt. Jamie's test, I'm sure, is more accurate than most, but inevitably it's still not 100%.

There's no doubt that we are going to see a lot more genetic tests being sold in the future, tests which try to predict not only whether you are a responder/nonresponder when it comes to aerobic fitness, but also whether exercise is likely to improve your glucose tolerance or whether you have the genes that will ensure that weight lifting will lead to bigger muscles.

A few of these gene tests will be useful, while others are likely to be of very low predictive value.

Some scientists hate the idea of these tests, not only because of the potential hype, but also because they fear that if they become widely available and people discover that they are nonresponders they will simply give up all exercise.

I think this is unlikely to happen because even if you are a nonresponder when it comes to one aspect of exercise, hopefully you are going to be a responder for another. I'm clearly never going to be a record-breaking long-distance runner but I am pleased that exercise has such a beneficial effect on my insulin. And, despite being something of an exercise-phobe, I have discovered that regular FastExercise makes me feel good and helps me keep the weight off.

Anyway, the upside to having a test which tells 20% of

the population that they are nonresponders is that the same tests will tell most people that they are responders and a lucky few (around 20% of the population) that if they take up exercise they are going to get enormous benefit. Peta, for example, was always likely to be a superresponder with an impressively large VO2 max (see page 360 for her score).

Peta's DNA Profile

Like Michael, I entered into the world of fitness DNA testing with some skepticism. As a lifelong exerciser what, I wondered, would the results reveal that I didn't already know?

Experience told me that I would probably be a responder. I've always found exercise not just easy but rewarding. While I knew I wasn't born with the "fast twitch muscle fibers" that would make me a good sprinter, hockey player, or jumper, and that I didn't have the genetic build that would allow me to bulk up with lots of weight training, I have always enjoyed endurance training such as long-distance running.

There are several companies that offer DNA testing. I tried two of the more established ones, with interesting results. The first suggested I was indeed a high-aerobic responder, best suited to endurance-type activities—a conclusion which fits perfectly with my fitness background.

But when I sent a swab off to the second company, they told me that my endurance potential was low and my abilities were much better suited to power and strength activities such as sprinting, weight training, and sports such as netball and football—for none of which, I might add, I have ever displayed the remotest bit of enthusiasm or aptitude. It could be, of course, that I have hidden talents and have missed sporting opportunities as a result of not knowing my genetic weaknesses. But I don't think so.

Clearly, the development of DNA tests is in its infancy and they are not yet completely reliable—hence my contradictory results. Still, if, as in Michael's case, they can help explain shortcomings and encourage you to focus your workouts more effectively, these tests certainly have a role to play. They have the potential to become a useful tool, helping us understand how individuals respond to exercise in starkly different ways.

Is HIT Safe?

With any form of exercise there is a risk that you will cause yourself some damage, particularly if you are not fit. The most common injuries are pulled muscles—which, as we all know, are easily incurred.

I have been to a few school sports days, particularly when my children were young, where the organizers have unwisely decided to include a "Fathers' Race." We fathers sheepishly volunteer, trying to look cool but secretly either dreading failure or hoping desperately to win. Some of the more competitive dads come in spiked training shoes; most of us come unprepared. We line up, our kids watching, keen not to disappoint. There is a shout, "go," and we sprint off faster than is wise.

Ten strides in and at least one of the dads is down, as if shot, clutching a hamstring or possibly his groin. I know this situation, I speak from personal experience, I have been there, done it, lain screaming on the ground calling for ice.

While pulling a muscle is painful, it is certainly not fatal. The real fear is that if you are unfit and then begin to do vigorous exercise the unexpected shock will lead to a heart attack or stroke. And this fear is magnified twentyfold when people think about HIT. They imagine a sweaty, overweight man in Lycra with clogged-up arteries getting onto his bike and, wham, a few strokes in, his flabby overworked heart packs up, leaving behind a grieving family.

So is this fear justified? As you'll see in Chapter 6, FastExercise: The Workouts, we suggest that if you are unfit you should ease yourself into HIT. I would also always recommend that anyone who has any doubts about their health should have a medical checkup before starting any form of exercise.

One of the factors that could trigger a heart attack or stroke is a dramatic rise in blood pressure. This is more likely to happen if you are doing something like weight training than if you are doing aerobic exercise. Your heart rate rises quite dramatically while doing HIT and that could put strain on the heart, which is why it is important to build up the amount of HIT you do over a period of time, allowing your body time to adjust.

In my view, though, the most compelling reason for believing that HIT is safe, even in the elderly or unfit, is that it has been tested on precisely those people who are most at risk of having a heart attack: people who have previously had one.

HIT and the Heart: Overturning Accepted Wisdom

When I was a medical student the accepted wisdom was that people who had had a heart attack and survived should take it easy. They were told to lie in bed, rest the heart, recover. Textbooks from the mid-1980s state unequivocally that "reduced activity is critical in patients with heart failure." This made perfect sense at the time—after all, if you'd had a near-fatal shock then surely rest was what was needed.

Then medical researchers did large-scale randomized trials and began to realize that this was not the best advice.

Trials like HF-ACTION, published in 2009,[12] showed that your chances of dying were significantly greater if you took to your bed. Common sense turned out to be wrong and now accepted wisdom has been turned on its head. These days doctors will advise you to mobilize as soon as possible, get back on your feet and get moving, often within days of your heart attack.

There has, therefore, been a paradigm shift, and I suspect

that this shift will, in time, also embrace HIT. Over the last decade a number of trials have been carried out in different countries looking at the risks and benefits of HIT in those with heart disease, and HIT always comes out well.

In a Norwegian study,[13] researchers compared the risks of having a heart attack or stroke after doing HIT or moderate-intensity training in a group of high-risk patients.

They took 4,846 patients with coronary heart disease from rehabilitation centers and randomly allocated them either to moderate-intensity training or to HIT. The patients who did moderate training, such as walking or jogging, put in a total of 129,456 hours of exercise. The HIT group did their exercise more intensely, but put in far fewer hours, a total of 46,364.

During a grand total of 175,820 hours of training in this high-risk group of patients there was one fatal heart attack. This was in the moderate training group. There were also two nonfatal heart attacks, in the HIT group.

The researchers' conclusion was that the risks of moderate or intense exercise are low, even in those with existing heart disease, and that "considering the significant cardiovascular adaptations associated with high-intensity exercise, such exercise should be considered among patients with coronary heart disease."

Similarly, in a review paper from 2012, "High-intensity interval training in cardiac rehabilitation," the authors looked at all the studies they could find that tested HIT in patients with coronary artery disease or heart failure. They concluded that "HIT appears to be safe and better tolerated by patients than moderate intensity continuous exercise (MICE)."

They go on to say that it is superior to standard exercise when it comes to producing improvements in heart function and quality of life.

Most recently a review paper from February 2013,[14] "High-intensity aerobic exercise in chronic heart failure," came to a similar conclusion: "High-intensity interval training is more effective than moderate intensity continuous exercise (MICE) for improving exercise capacity in patients with heart failure."

Clearly, more research is required, but what I take from the studies done so far is that HIT—in fact any form of aerobic exercise—is more likely to cut your risk of having a heart attack or stroke than cause you to have one.

If you have any health concerns, see your doctor. Otherwise it's time to get your trainers on. In the next chapter, Peta will put you through your paces.

CHAPTER SIX

FastExercise: The Workouts

THE GREAT THING ABOUT FASTEXERCISE IS THAT IT can be worked into a busy life with relative ease. It's less of a full-time commitment, more of an addition to the way you live. You can, if you really want, do FastExercise in your normal clothes, not even bothering to change into trainers, let alone gym gear. It's not something I do, but it is something Michael does. The fact it can be done in a suit or skirt without breaking sweat demonstrates how easily FastExercise workouts can be slotted into your day.

The other appealing thing about FastExercise is that it encompasses many different approaches, which is good because it's important to vary the way you exercise. Variety ensures you are kept on your toes, your body and mind never knowing what you are going to throw at them next.

Under the FastExercise umbrella we have included two types of exercise with very different purposes—FastFitness and FastStrength. Both are extremely time efficient. Within these two categories, we have also included a range of different plans. Find the one that suits you, but try also to vary them.

FastFitness is based on HIT, the aim being to boost your cardiovascular system and reduce your diabetes risk.

For good muscle tone and flexibility, however, we also suggest FastStrength. These exercises strengthen the major muscle groups and rely on your body weight to achieve results. They can be done in a few minutes, without any special equipment, at home, at work, in a hotel room (all you need is a chair and tolerant neighbors) or while out for a run or walk (in which case you will need an empty park bench).

Depending on how long you want to spend warming up or cooling down, most FastFitness or FastStrength exercises can be done in less than ten minutes a day or just incorporated into what you are already doing.

The rule with HIT, or FastFitness, is to try and do three sessions a week, either as part of another exercise regime (e.g., add HIT to your run), as part of your commute (Michael often does it on his bike traveling home), or by itself. The temptation will probably be to do more. Don't. It won't make it more effective and the danger is, if you go crazy, you'll damage yourself.

When it comes to FastStrength exercises, the rules are more flexible. Jamie Timmons works on his main muscle groups three times a week on days when he is not doing HIT. Michael likes to do them more often, up to five times a week. As do I, and I also vary my regime quite a bit—on nice days getting out to do a quick session in my local park (see the Park Workout on page 322). Ideally, the FastStrength exercises should be done on nonconsecutive days—so a maximum of three days a week. Try to vary the mix so that you work as many different body parts as you can.

Aim to split your time about 50–50 between FastFitness and FastStrength, and you won't go far wrong. A typical weekly program for the average exerciser, therefore, might comprise two days of FastFitness, two days of FastStrength; and a typical week for those who are fitter and keener, say three days of FastFitness and two days of FastStrength.

Before You Get Going . . .

Warm-up and cooldown: how much, if any, is necessary?

These are the bookends of any workout, the fitness components that promise to reduce injuries and fight fatigue. But are lengthy warm-ups and cooldowns as essential as every personal trainer would have us believe?

The Warm-up

When it comes to HIT, most studies are based on a warm-up of 2–5 minutes of gentle, workout-specific activity (so, walking or running if you are sprinting, cycling if you are Fast Exercising on a bike, swimming if you are in the pool). Some researchers think you need less. There are no clear rules.

Michael warms up in just one minute for his cycle sessions, sometimes less. I prefer 5–10 minutes for running workouts. A warm-up should literally heat the body to increase blood flow, and loosen the muscles to ensure they are ready for activity. Warm muscles pull oxygen from the bloodstream more easily and trigger the chemical reactions needed to produce energy more efficiently. None of the workouts that are outlined on the pages that follow should be started without any preparation; how much is largely up to you.

Stretching

It's widely believed that static stretching—the kind that involves holding a movement, such as bending over and touching your toes—makes your muscles more flexible, primes them for activity, and reduces the chance of injury. That belief, widespread though it is, doesn't seem to be based on hard evidence. Indeed, the kind of stretches most of us think we should do before exercise—touching the toes or extending the hamstrings—have no obvious advantages and may be detrimental.

When Dr. Ian Shrier, of the Centre for Epidemiology at the Jewish General Hospital in Montreal, reviewed the evidence on preworkout stretching for *The Physician and Sports Medicine Journal* several years ago,[1] he found that stretching immediately before a gym session actually led to a reduction in muscle power. The effects were small and temporary, but significant enough for Shrier, a past president of the Canadian Academy of Sport and Exercise Medicine, to recommend dropping stretches from warm-ups.

There is also the question of whether stretching reduces injuries. Most studies suggest it doesn't. A review article in

Sports Medicine[2] makes the sensible point that if the sport you are doing involves a lot of stop-start (e.g., football) then you might get some benefit from stretching; but if you are running, jogging, or swimming, there is strong evidence that stretching has "no beneficial effect on injury prevention."

If you want to stretch before you start, make it dynamic, with movements such as arm circling and sidestepping. Dynamic movements send a message from the brain to the muscles saying, "We are ready to work out." Static stretching, by contrast, triggers an inhibitory response in the brain. For sports like football, dynamic stretching might mean a bit of ball kicking and dribbling.

The Cooldown

Much less research has been conducted on the value of the cooldown and the research that has been done has produced little evidence either way. After a burst of intense exercise it is best not to stop moving entirely. When you work out really hard, the heart has to pump much faster, and blood vessels expand, leading to greater blood flow to the legs and feet. If you stop too suddenly, blood can start to pool in the lower limbs, causing dizziness.

Michael gets his HIT mainly from cycling and he spends about a minute doing gentle cycling after a fierce burst to allow his blood pressure and heart rate to return to normal. I, on the other hand, like to spend at least five minutes after a FastExercise workout doing the same activity at a slower pace. I find it brings everything back to equilibrium.

The Dreaded DOMS (Delayed Onset Muscle Soreness)

Another popular myth is that cooldown stretches will stop your muscles from becoming sore by flushing out lactic acid, one of the so-called waste products of exercise. Some gym instructors will tell you that it is the buildup of lactic acid that makes your muscles tired. This is nonsense.

Yes, strenuous exercise will lead to greater production of lactic acid but the reason this happens is because lactate is needed as a fuel. Without it you wouldn't be able to push yourself as hard as you do.

The soreness you get after exercise isn't caused by a buildup of lactic acid, but by minor damage to muscle fibers, and stretching will have no effect on that. The only real remedy is rest.

In an Australian study, in which volunteers were asked to walk backwards on a treadmill for half an hour to induce calf-muscle stiffness,[3] researchers found that doing a warm-up made a small difference to perceived muscle soreness two days later but a ten-minute cooldown made no difference. Personally, I like to stretch at the end of the day. It helps me to relax and to unknot the tensions of the day. But find what works for you.

Painkillers

A word of warning. You might be tempted to take anti-inflammatory agents like aspirin or ibuprofen before doing exercise to reduce muscle soreness afterwards. Don't. Numerous studies have shown that they won't reduce muscle soreness and that they can cause bleeding in the stomach and gastrointestinal leakage, bacteria getting out of your gut and into your blood.

And Finally, Before You Start: Keeping Track

We recommend you keep track of your progress in an exercise diary. The kinds of measurements you might record once a month or so could include:

* ★ Strength—how many push-ups can you comfortably do?

* ★ Resting heart rate

* ★ Weight and waist measurement

* ★ Your aerobic fitness, as measured by your VO2 max

* ★ Your glucose tolerance

To find out how to do these, see the section on measuring the impact of exercise at the back of the book.

FastFitness—Ways to Get Your HIT

There are all sorts of activities that will enable you to get the intensity required for FastFitness. The following six are ordered according to the likely level of benefit revealed by research, but also according to our personal preference. Cycling is first because it is how most HIT studies have been done so far, and it's Michael's favorite (though he's partial to stair running, too). Running comes next because it is a popular form of exercise, good for HIT, and it is my preferred way; cross-training is Jamie Timmons's favorite, also a good all-around form of training for those who prefer to work out in a gym. Of the rest, I would say that they are all good forms of exercise in themselves, but less is known about their particular suitability for HIT—and be careful with rowing, which has the potential to cause injury with poor technique.

Cycling

Indoor cycling is a good way of getting HIT because a modern indoor bike lets you add resistance, changing the intensity of the ride. It also enables you to continue exercising when it's cold, wet, and dark outside. And, unlike some other forms of exercise, it is less prone to cause injuries. Most of the academic studies on HIT have involved volunteers using special indoor stationary bikes because they are well suited to laboratory studies. However, many people prefer the fresh air and unpredictable terrain they encounter outside. On a road or mountain bike the exercise intensity can be altered by switching to a higher gear and by cycling hard uphill. Wind can also add resistance, making an outdoor cycle more intense. As we will see in the next few pages, the duration of sprints can vary from twenty seconds to four minutes depending on which FastFitness session you

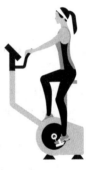

choose. Indoor bikes should be set at a minimum of 90 rpm, gradually working towards a cycling speed of 110 rpm as you get fitter and stronger.

Running

Running (or jogging) requires no special equipment, other than a pair of trainers, a T-shirt, and some shorts. It can be done almost anywhere and offers clear health benefits in its own right.

To make a normal run into HIT you will have to inject intensity into your workout, which means you need to throw in a few sprints, preferably up a hill. By pushing your body on an incline you are working your muscles much harder than when you run on the flat. A hill should be challenging but not so steep that you can't run up it fast. If you are not especially fit, build up to this gradually.

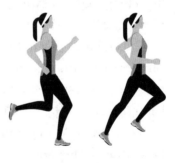

Start by trying to run flat out up a hill for ten seconds. As you get fitter, build slowly up to, say, 30 seconds. After running up a hill you should avoid jogging back down; walk down instead.

Use natural markers (trees, lampposts) to establish distances, or a stopwatch to time your sprints. Try to vary the terrain on which you run—grass, dirt trails, running tracks, and pavements are all suitable.

Running well uphill requires rhythm: shorten your stride slightly compared to when you are running on the flat and aim to keep your leg turnover constant. Don't lean forward from the waist or back—your head, shoulders, and back should form a straight line over your feet.

Running on a Treadmill

There are two kinds of runners: those who like treadmills and those who don't. Personally, I can't see the appeal of the hamster-wheel confinement of a mechanical running belt, but many people find the treadmill reassuringly familiar. Nothing ever changes—no wind, no rain, no traffic—so they know exactly what to expect.

When it comes to performing HIT on a treadmill, the major downside is having to deal with the mechanics. Switching speeds between the desired intensity for HIT and recovery can be tricky and is almost never instant. Studies have also shown that indoor running burns about 5% fewer calories than running outdoors, partly because of the lack of wind resistance and partly because the treadmill's motorized belt propels you slightly. For these reasons, it's advisable to crank up the gradient in order to make sure you are working hard enough. Research at the University of Brighton suggests treadmill users who want to achieve the same workload intensity as running on flat terrain outdoors need to set the machine at a permanent 1% incline.

Again the time spent on a treadmill varies according to which session you choose to follow. The key to doing FastExercise on a treadmill is to increase the gradient so that you are forced to work harder. It's quite tricky to do FastExercise well on a treadmill because of the time lapse when switching from fast to slow running during the recovery. It's much harder to run fast up a hill and it will save drastic changes in speed settings.

Stair Running

If you have access to several flights of stairs, either at work or at home, they constitute a terrific HIT circuit. The American Lung Association says that stair running provides the same benefits as conventional running in half the time, because you are constantly working against gravity. Stair running is fairly low impact on the knees and feet and is one of the best activities for bottom and leg toning. Make sure you use good technique: don't hunch your back or twist your head, and bend your arms at right angles to provide power as they pump. Make sure that your whole foot lands on each step, to avoid straining the Achilles tendon— and walk (don't run) back downstairs during recovery periods. Or take the lift. As with all FastExercise, the key is to move fast. Sprint hard up the stairs, let your legs feel the burn, and slowly recover on the way back down.

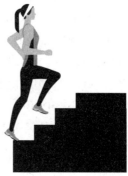

Cross-Training

With a cross-trainer you can work lots of different muscles in a short period of time. Set it on the highest incline and resistance. Gently move your arms and legs for one minute to loosen up. Then pick up the tempo, aiming to give a maximum effort (high tempo) for about 30 seconds, before slowing down.

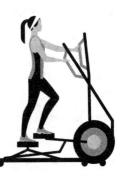

Swimming

It is the natural resistance of water that makes swimming physically challenging, and the faster you try to swim, the harder you are going to have to work. Swimming uses a lot of muscles but it is important to occasionally vary the strokes. Rather than judging things by time it may be easier to judge by distance. A 25-meter length at full speed is comparable to sprinting for around 30–40 seconds. Start by swimming as fast as you can for 25 meters in around twenty seconds, gradually increasing your speed as you get fitter.

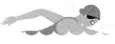

Rowing

An indoor rowing machine will, like a cross-trainer, work the entire body and be extremely challenging, but it is one of those pieces of equipment you need to be wary of as you can hurt yourself quite badly if you don't know what you are doing. Good technique is crucial. Start each stroke by pushing with the legs, not pulling with the arms, and keep your wrists in line with the handle so that the pulley wire is parallel to the floor. Make sure your back is straight, not rounded, to increase the power of each stroke and reduce the pressure on your lower back. 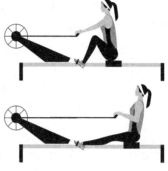 Since rowing engages muscles in the whole body, it is relatively easy to hit high intensities on the go. To sprint, increase your stroke rate, then recover by slowing it to what seems like a "resting" level.

Jump Rope

Jumping rope, like running, is convenient. However, it's quite hard to involve lots of muscle groups and achieve the necessary intensity. Avoid buying traditional woven ropes as these are heavy (even more so when wet) and slow to turn. Ball bearings and jump counters also add unnecessary weight and make ropes more cumbersome. Your best bet is a lightweight, flexible plastic or leather gymnastic "speed" rope. Knees and ankles should be flexed but your torso kept straight when jumping. Arms should be at your side with the rope turning from the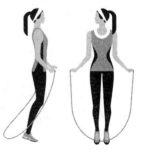

wrists and forearms. It can be helpful to set your stopwatch or a timer that beeps to let you know when to start jumping faster and harder.

The Workouts

In the next few pages, I outline a variety of FastFitness workouts. Between us Michael and I have tried and tested every variation on the theme. We each have our favorites among the suggestions below. And we each have those that we feel are bringing benefit even if we don't always relish the prospect of completing them. Just remember: the discomfort (and there should be an element of puffing, panting, muscle soreness, and all-over fatigue) is temporary. In less than the time it takes to drive to the gym it will all be over.

The following workouts should ideally be done 2–3 times a week. We have ordered them roughly in terms of the amount of time you spend doing the intense part of the exercise. The total amount of time you actually spend on each workout will depend on a number of factors, including how long you choose to warm up and cool down.

The actual intensity of the exercise is up to you; wearing a heart-rate monitor will give you an indication of how hard you are pushing yourself, but the important thing is to start slowly and build up gradually so your body has time to adapt. Don't overdo it on the first day.

The Bare Minimum

40 seconds' hard exercise (2 x 20 seconds)
Total—4–6 minutes, including recovery

Unbelievably, there is evidence that just 40 seconds of intense activity can make a difference. In 2011 Dr. Niels Vollaard and colleagues at Bath University did a study[4] in which they asked fifteen healthy but sedentary young men and women to try something they called REHIT (reduced-exertion high-intensity training) for six weeks.

He started them off in the first week with a couple of minutes of gentle cycling, then one 10-second burst of intense cycling followed by a couple of minutes of cooldown. In weeks two and three, each exercise session consisted of a warm-up, fifteen seconds of all-out sprinting, a couple of minutes of recovery, another fifteen seconds of all-out sprinting, then the gentle cooldown.

For the final three weeks they cranked it up so each exercise session consisted of two 20-second flat-out sprints separated by a couple of minutes of recovery.

Despite the fact that over the six weeks the volunteers had done less than ten minutes of hard exercise, both the men and the women showed significant improvements in their aerobic fitness (VO2 max up 15% and 12% respectively). When it came to insulin sensitivity, there was a gender difference: the men's improved by 28% while the women's did not improve.

Niels is currently carrying out further studies to see if this gender difference is real and also to see if people with metabolic syndrome and diabetes get similar improvements.

He is also keen, at some point, to see if a single burst of twenty seconds done three times a week makes a measurable difference. If you are only doing a few bursts twenty seconds seems to be the minimum time for a burst that will make a difference.

The basic principle here is to push yourself in two brief 20-second bursts. The most obvious activity to choose is cycling, since that was what they did in the trials; if you are doing it indoors, you will need an exercise bike with variable resistance on which you can crank up the intensity mechanically; and, if cycling outside, you will need to find a hill, preferably quite a steep one, and use gravity to increase your workload. But in principle, any of the activities above will work fine. In the case of running, you will need to find some way of cranking up the resistance for your 20-second spurts—either mechanically, on a treadmill in the gym, or by using a hill if you are outside.

★ Start off with a couple of minutes of gentle pedaling/running/swimming.

★ When you feel ready, speed up and work your body as hard as you can for twenty seconds, before slowing down.

★ Repeat the sprint after you've had a couple of minutes of gentle pedaling/jogging/walking to recover. Recovery time is important.

In total the Bare Minimum should take less than ten minutes. Michael likes to do it on an exercise bike (see box below) and, now that he's more used to it, he does it in less than four minutes by minimizing warm-up and cooldown and by cutting his gentle pedaling to about a minute.

If you are very unfit or have never tried HIT before, it may be worth slowly building up the sprints from 2 x 10 seconds to 2 x 20 seconds. Once you have mastered 2 x 20 seconds you may want to add on another 20-second sprint which, along with the recommended recovery period, will add another couple of minutes to your regime.

How Michael Does It

1. Put the kettle on.
2. Get on the exercise bike and do a couple of minutes of gentle cycling, against limited resistance. You should just about notice the effort in your thighs.
3. After about two minutes begin pedaling fast, then swiftly crank up the resistance.
4. The amount of resistance you select will depend on your current strength and fitness. It should be high enough that

after fifteen seconds of sprinting your thighs begin to burn and the speed at which you are pedaling slows, simply because your muscles are fatigued and you cannot keep going at that pace.

5. If, after fifteen seconds, you can still keep going at the same pace then the resistance you've chosen is not quite high enough. It mustn't, however, be so high that you grind to a complete halt. It's a matter of experimenting. What you'll find is that as you get fitter the amount of resistance you can cope with increases. It is important that you keep increasing the resistance to ensure each 20-second work-out involves maximum effort.

6. After your first burst of fast sprinting, drop the resistance and do a couple of minutes of gentle pedaling to catch your breath and let your muscles recharge.

7. Then, when you feel ready, do another 20-second burst.

8. Relax! It's over! Finish with a couple of minutes of gentle cycling to allow your heart rate and blood pressure to return to normal before stepping off the bike and having a cup of tea.

How Peta Gets Her 20-Second HIT While Running

The Bare Minimum workout doesn't have to be a stand-alone session. I prefer to weave it into a slightly longer run or walk of 15–20 minutes rather than head to the park for just 40 seconds of exercise. My approach is to run at a moderate pace for 5–10 minutes and then perform the lung-burning 20-second flat-out burst. I then jog for another 3–4 minutes before doing the second sprint and finish with a 5-minute gentle run. Those short bursts are tougher than you might think. If you do them properly with pumping arms and fast leg speed, you will feel your thighs burn and your heart rate soar after each one—which is a positive thing. Personally, I like to do the sprints around the edge of a football or cricket field so that I can try to get a bit farther each time I do it. But fit them in when and where you can—even on the walk to school or work.

How to Do the Bare Minimum at Work

FastExercise can be done at work, whether your employer provides a gym or not, as long as you work somewhere with at least four flights of stairs.

You can do this regime in a suit, but if you wear high heels you will need to replace them with more sensible flat rubber-soled shoes.

First find a quiet stairwell in a building with at least four full floors. If you are unfit, you may want to spend a few weeks walking up the four flights before attempting anything more adventurous.

When you feel up to it, try bounding up the stairs for twenty seconds. And I mean *bounding*. If you are a beginner, this should be long enough to make you breathe heavily and to feel the buildup of fatigue in your thighs. As you get fitter you will find that you need to run for longer, up more stairs, to get the same feeling.

Ideally take the lift down to where you started, or in a tall building just pause for 1–2 minutes to catch your breath before bounding up another few floors.

The 30-Second Sprinter

2 minutes' hard exercise
Total—16 minutes, including 14 minutes' recovery

This is similar to the 20-second sprints that we have just described, except that you will need a longer recovery period between sprints because going from twenty seconds to thirty seconds of all-out sprinting is much more demanding.

If you are not used to HIT, you should start gradually, preferably by working your way through a 20-second regime first, then trying 2 x 30 seconds and building up from there.

Make time to do a couple of minutes of warm-up and ensure you are mentally ready before starting your first sprint. Between each sprint pedal gently for 3–4 minutes to recover (you will need it).

This regime is based on the original HIT studies, which were done in Canada and were called SIT (sprint interval training). The Canadians found that doing four 30-second sprints (interspersed with a few minutes of recovery) three times a week led to similar improvements in fitness as running or cycling at a steady speed for many hours a week.[5]

30-second sprint/bike: 4 x 30-second sprints on a bike. Make time to do a couple of minutes' warm-up before starting your first sprint. Between each sprint take 3–4 minutes to recover by pedaling at a gentle pace (you will need it). Then take at least 2 minutes to cool down.

30-second sprint/run: 4 x 30-second running sprints up a hill. Warm up by running at a gentle pace to your chosen hill. Then sprint for 30 seconds up the hill; walk down or around for a few minutes, then do it again. And again. And again. Finish by jogging slowly home. Stretch if you like.

30-second sprint/swim: If you like swimming, do the first few lengths at a gentle pace. When you are ready, try swimming 25 meters flat out (or count to 30 in your head). Take a bit of a breather, then continue gently swimming a couple more lengths. Then do another sprint. Repeat four times. Finish with a very gentle couple of lengths.

The 60-Second Workout

2½ minutes' hard exercise
Total—10–11 minutes, including 8 minutes' recovery

This is one of my favorite approaches and a format I have used for many years. It's very simple: the basic principle is to alternate 60-second bursts of activity with 90-second recovery periods—for example, 1 minute on, 1½ minutes off. It's wonderfully flexible: it can be done with any of the activities listed above, like cycling, running, swimming, and can be scaled down or up according to what you require.

You might think that 60 seconds of HIT has to be tougher than 30 seconds, but this version is not. The 60-second workout evolved out of work done by the sports science team at McMaster University when they were trying to find an effective but "gentler" version of the challenging 30-Second Sprinter. The key difference is that you don't push yourself quite as hard. Instead of going flat-out, you exercise for a minute at about 90% of your best effort, aiming to push your heart rate up to around 80% of HR max (see section on measuring the impact of exercise at the back of the book) by the end of the first minute. (To find out your HR max, see the reference section at the back.)

In the original studies they asked the volunteers to do 10 x 1-minute bursts of HIT with 90 seconds recovery in between each burst. This is what I do. More recently researchers from Metapredict (a group of exercise academics) have begun testing a less demanding variant, involving a maximum of 5 x 60-second bursts alternated with 90-second recovery periods.

The less fit should definitely start with three bursts; if you are superkeen, and really want to push your limits, you can do the full 10 (this is effectively the Roger Bannister version, and particularly beneficial if you are preparing for an endurance event). Our recommendation, if you are basically quite fit, is that you aim for a steady five. So:

★ Two minutes of warm-up.

★ 5 x 60-second bursts of activity, with 90 seconds' recovery between each burst.

★ One minute of cooldown.

The Fat Burner

8 minutes' hard exercise
Total—20 minutes, including 12 minutes' recovery

This workout involves a repetitive cycle of eight seconds of intense activity alternated with twelve seconds of recovery, and is only really suitable for an exercise bike. It is based on two key Australian studies by Stephen Boutcher,[6] which showed that HIT could lead to significant fat loss.

After a brief warm-up, you cycle hard against resistance for eight seconds, then gently for twelve, then hard against resistance again for eight seconds, and gently for twelve, and so on.

To begin with, you maintain this pattern for about five minutes. The aim, as you get fitter, is to build up to fifteen or even twenty minutes. The resistance stays constant throughout the twenty minutes, high enough so it feels strenuous. Gradually build up resistance over the first few weeks.

The Four-Minute Sprinter

Total—4 minutes' hard exercise

This is different because, instead of exerting yourself in intervals, you are doing it all in one go. Norwegian researchers found that a single four-minute burst of running/jogging/walking on a treadmill at a hard pace done three times a week was enough to boost the health and fitness of previously sedentary middle-aged men significantly. At the end of their ten-week trial the men had improved their aerobic capacity by 10% or more, lost a couple of pounds of fat, lowered their blood pressure, and had better blood sugar control.[7]

Four-minute sprinter/bike: After a warm-up, do four minutes of hard cycling at around 90% of maximal effort.

Four-minute sprinter/run: After a warm-up, do a four-minute run at 90% of your maximum pace (this will leave you tired and breathless. You should definitely not be chatting). An alternative is to see how far you can run in four minutes—and try to better it next time. Do it in the local park, using markers such as trees or posts. Or try it on an athletics track.

Four-minute sprinter/stair sprint: Run hard up a flight of stairs and walk back down the same flight, covering as many "fast" flights as possible in four minutes. As you get fitter, try to increase the number of flights you can manage in the time span. You should be able to manage about 10 flights.

Four-minute sprinter/walk: The researchers recommend a brisk four-minute walk uphill at an 8–10% gradient (this is quite steep), perhaps to or from work.

FastWalking

This is a great staple, which can be built easily into your day—your walk to work, to and from the local shops—and is surprisingly effective. Walking up a hill, fast enough to get your pulse racing, is ideal but it can also be done on the flat. Like other forms of FastExercise, FastWalking (where you alternate fast with slow) seems to have more impact than ordinary low-intensity strolling. The studies I've seen (see pages 351–352) show that it leads to more fat loss, improved fitness, and glucose control. The studies are based on walking fast in three-minute bursts. If you're not fit, then aim for something more modest, like 1–2 minutes.

★ Begin by walking at a normal pace, just to warm up.

★ When you are ready, pick up the pace. On the RPE (rate of perceived exertion) scale where 1 is light and 10 is very hard, you should be aiming at 6–7— it should be hard, but you should be able to keep going. Then slow down and give yourself at least three minutes of slower walking to recover.

★ Repeat a couple of times.

★ Start off by trying a twenty-minute FastWalk a couple of times a week. As you get fitter, increase the length of the walk and the number of times you put in a Fast burst.

FastStrength—Working with Your Body Weight

For maximum health gains, you need to exercise not only your heart and lungs but also other major muscle groups. FastStrength is a form of circuit training, except it can be done at home without special equipment and it is best done fast. The idea is to exercise as many major muscle groups as possible, and to alternate between activities in such a way as to give the ones not being worked a bit of a rest. So, if you are doing push-ups (working the upper body), you should follow these with an activity that works the core (say, abdominal crunches) or the legs (squats).

Similarly, if you've just done a workout that produces a big increase in heart rate, such as jumping jacks, the next exercise should be one that is more sedate, such as a wall sit.

To pack it all into as little time as possible and to maximize metabolic impact you should do as many repeats of each exercise as you can manage in 30 seconds and take just 10 seconds' rest between each.

The FastStrength approach is based on a paper in the *American College of Sports Medicine's Health & Fitness Journal*[8] and is now one of Michael's favorite regimes.

This approach is designed to combine aerobic and resistance training and it can, as the song says, be done anytime, anywhere. Although you should start by doing one 7-minute session twice a week, as you get fitter you may want to fit in another session, and also vary the exercises. Ideally you should do around three FastStrength sessions a week on nonconsecutive days.

There is nothing new about the exercises that are recommended in the paper, just the way the combinations are put together.

A note of caution: if you have elevated blood pressure (hypertension), it is best to avoid isometric exercises like the wall sit, the side plank, and the plank.

Suggested exercises:

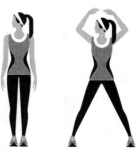

Jumping Jacks
Stand with your hands by your sides. In one movement, jump up, spreading your legs apart as you raise your arms over your head. You

should land with your arms over your head and your feet more than hip-width apart. Jump up again and in one movement, bring your legs together and your arms back to your sides. The jumping jacks should be fast, but controlled. You have just done one jumping jack. Keep going for 30 seconds.

Push-ups

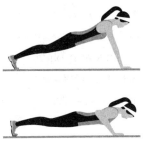

Lie facedown with the palms of your hands directly beneath your shoulders and the balls of your feet touching the ground. Keep your body straight—your head in line with your back—and raise yourself up using your arms. Lower your torso to the ground until your elbows form a 90-degree angle and then push up again. If you find this too hard, perform the exercise with your knees on the ground until you are strong enough to do the full thing. Record how many you can do in 30 seconds. These should be done in a fast, but controlled manner.

Wall Sit

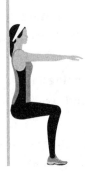

Start with your back against a wall with your feet shoulder-width apart and positioned about two feet from the wall. Slowly slide your back down the wall until your thighs are parallel with the ground. Adjust your feet if you need to so that your knees are directly above your ankles (rather than over your toes). Don't arch your back. Hold this position, if you can, for 30 seconds. Rest ten seconds between sets.

Abdominal Crunches

Lie on your back with your knees bent and feet flat on the floor and your hands positioned by your sides (or lightly at the sides of your head). Curl up your upper body without lifting your lower back off the floor. Make sure your chin is tucked in to- 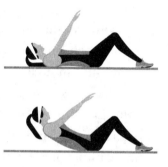 wards your chest. When your shoulders and upper back are lifted off the floor, curl back down. Again, it's 30 seconds, and these should be done in a fast, but controlled manner.

Step-ups on a Chair

Use a bench or sturdy chair with a seat that is at a comfortable height to step onto. Place one foot on the "step," making sure your whole foot is in contact with the surface. Push your body weight up, driving your weight through your heel and breathing out as you do this, until you are standing on top of the step with both feet. Step back and down, one leg at a time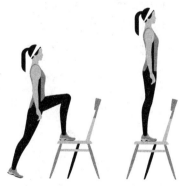

until you are standing with both feet flat on the floor again. Repeat with the opposite leg leading. Step-ups should be performed with care but at a brisk pace, for—you guessed it—30 seconds.

Squats

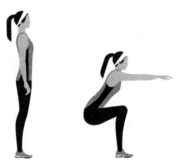

Stand with feet shoulder-width apart and hands placed lightly on opposite shoulders. Bend from the hips, keeping the weight in your heels. Make sure your back is straight. Keep bending until your legs are at a 90-degree angle—imagine you are preparing to sit in a chair. Push back up without bending your back. These should be done in a steady and controlled fashion.

Tricep Dips

Stand with your back to a bench or chair; place your palms on the seat behind you, bending your knees at right angles, hips straight. Bend your elbows to 90 degrees to lower your body (so that your bottom descends halfway to the floor).

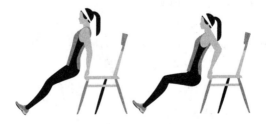

Push yourself back up using only your arms. These exercises should be done quickly, but with control.

Plank

Lie on the floor and then raise yourself onto your forearms and toes so that your body forms a straight line from head to toe. Make sure your midsection doesn't rise or drop. Squeeze your buttocks and hold the position for as long as possible. Remember, this exercise should never cause pain in the lower back. The first time you try this you probably won't manage 30 seconds. Do what you can, and if you can't hold for 30 seconds, try 10 seconds, resting for 5 and holding for 10, for a total of 30 seconds.

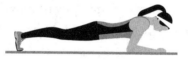

High-knee Running

Stand tall and begin jogging either on the spot or forward. Without leaning back, drive through the balls of your feet and try to bring your knees close to chest level. Keep your hands relaxed, elbows bent and shoulders down, and swing your arms back and forth to help you keep going. Again, 30 seconds of this is hard work. You can start slowly, but ideally these should be fast and high.

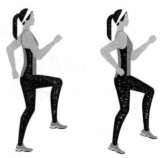

Lunge

Stand with your back straight and feet shoulder-width apart. Step forward with one leg, bending both knees to 90 degrees and keeping your upper body straight. Pull back to the starting position and repeat, putting the other leg forward. These should be done in a steady but controlled manner.

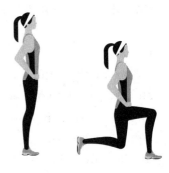

Push-up with Rotation

Assume the classic push-up position (see page 314), but as you straighten your arms in the upward move, rotate your body so that your right arm extends overhead. Your arms and torso should form a "T." Return to the starting position, lower yourself by bending your elbows, then push up and rotate till your left hand points towards the ceiling.

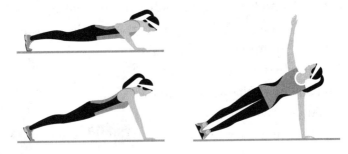

Side Plank

Lie on your side and raise your body so that your weight is supported by your lower forearm and feet. Maintain a diagonal line with your body, keeping your hips off the floor. Make sure your neck and back are straight. Hold for as long as possible—ideally 30 seconds. If you can't, try holding for 10 seconds, resting for 5, holding for 10—for a total of 30 seconds.

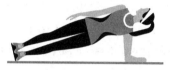

These are the basics. But there are lots of variants. For example, you could try a:

Plank with leg raise: Lie facedown with your elbows on the ground; elevate your body, keeping your weight distributed between your forearms and feet. Your elbows should be bent at a 90-degree angle. Keep your back straight with your hips raised off the floor. Squeeze your torso tight, slowly lifting one foot 6–8 inches off the ground, and hold the position for a few seconds. Lower your leg back to the starting position. Hold for as long as possible—ideally 30 seconds. If you can't, try holding for 10 seconds, resting for 5, holding for 10—for a total of 30 seconds.

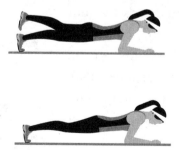

Side plank with reach around: Lie on your side and elevate your body, supporting your weight between your forearm and feet. Keep your body straight with your hips off the floor; your neck and back should stay straight. Raise your upper arm straight above you so that it's perpendicular to the floor. Reach under and behind your torso with that hand, then lift your arm back up to the starting position. Hold for as long as possible—ideally 30 seconds. If you can't, try holding for 10 seconds, resting for 5, holding for 10—for a total of 30 seconds.

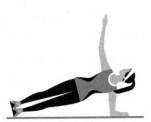

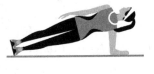

Reverse curl: as an alternative to the plank, lie on your back, with your hands by your sides, your feet up, and your thighs perpendicular to the floor. They should not go lower than this for the entire movement. Using your lower abs, roll your pelvis to raise your hips off the

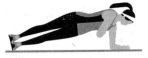

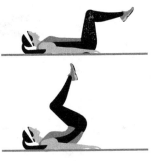

floor. Your legs will now be at a 45-degree angle to the floor. Hold briefly at top position. Return slowly to the start position. Repeat in a controlled way for 30 seconds.

Even Faster HIT

There are all sorts of ways you can mix up these particular exercises. The following circuits can all be done in just four minutes. Make sure you include variety so that your legs, arm, and trunk muscles are all worked.

Fast ladder: Choose four exercises from either of the lists above and do them ten times each, then nine times, then eight times—until you perform just one repetition of each. My preferred routine is:

★ Squats

★ Lunges

★ 10-meter sprint shuttle runs (back-to-back sprints). Only practical if you are outside.

★ Tricep dips

Fast max reps: Choose three of the body-weight (FastStrength) exercises listed above, do each one ten times. Move as fast as you possibly can to get through as many rounds as possible in four minutes.

The Park Workout

It might sound an odd admission for a fitness writer, but I'm no fan of gyms. I find the gym environment sterile and far from motivational; I feel self-conscious surrounded by mirrors and supertoned workout fanatics. Gym classes, too, leave me exasperated with their choreographed content and repetition. But most of all I miss being outdoors.

Exercise outside and your skin is kissed by the breeze. There is exposure to real, natural daylight that has untold benefits for mind and body—boosting your mood and vitamin D stores. Numerous studies have shown that outdoor or "green" exercise improves not only our daily mood but our general mental health. Researchers at the University of Essex showed that just five minutes of workouts in the park enhanced subjects' mental well-being, while other studies have shown that people who have exerted themselves outside have lower blood levels of cortisol, a hormone related to stress, than those who have exercised inside.

More than anything else, perhaps, there is an element of unpredictability that not only prevents you from getting bored, but actually helps you work harder. Studies have shown that exercising outdoors on undulating ground and changing surfaces, often with wind for added resistance, uses far more energy than slapping the soles of your trainers on the conveyor belt of a treadmill.

Of course, FastExercise is perfectly suited to be performed indoors or out, but for something different I like to throw the odd park circuit into the mix. Some of the bench exercises below are the brainchild of sports scientist Steve Mellor. Others are exercises I myself have found to be effective over the years. So, find a tree, a path, or a park bench and off you go.

Perform 10 repetitions of 2–4 of the exercises below, alternating them for a total of 3–6 minutes. Move as fast as you possibly can, and try and get through as many rounds as possible of the exercises in the time. For example, do 10 seconds of bear crawling, 30 seconds of mountain climber, and bench-up for 15 seconds. Then repeat the minicircuit as many times as you can for five minutes.

Bear Crawl

Put on some old clothes and head for the park. Start on all fours and begin moving along the ground as quickly as you can. Add variations—move the arm and leg from the same side of your body at the same time, or move the opposite arm and foot. Keep your hips straight and low at first (as if stalking something in a bush) and then change to a high-level crawl. Crawl for ten seconds.

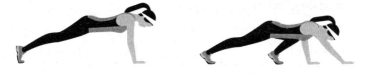

Log Haul

This is fine, again, if you don't mind getting dirty, and should only be performed with a log or rock that is not so heavy that it is a strain to lift it. Squat down from the knees (keeping your back straight) to pick up the item and lift it, preferably to shoulder level. If it's too heavy, carry it with your arms straight, keeping good spinal alignment. Carry it a distance of 10 meters, aiming to move as quickly as possible.

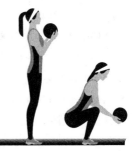

Deep Squat

Stand with your feet wider than hip-width apart and your back straight. Bend your knees to drop down into as deep a squat as possible with your buttocks aiming for the ground. The position should feel relaxed and you should keep

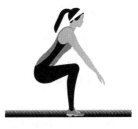

your heels on the ground. Allow your arms to hang in front of your body and keep your head in line with your spine. If you find this too difficult at first, try holding on to a bench or tree for support. Hold the position for fifteen seconds.

Mountain Climber

Facing a bench, place your hands on the edge of the seat and extend your legs behind you in a push-up position

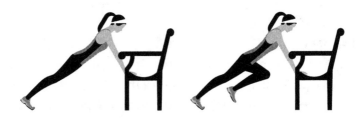

with head, back, and feet in a straight line. Drive one knee up in between the arms, then drive the foot back down into the start position and quickly change legs. Only one foot should be on the floor at any one time—aim to mimic a sprinting style.

Bench Push-up

Assume a plank position by placing your hands on the front edge of a bench, your body in a straight line, so that your weight is supported on the balls of your feet and by your elbows (bent to 90 degrees). Don't allow your back to arch, or your hips to drop. Push up until your arms are straight; then lower them back down so that both elbows are bent at 90 degrees. Repeat.

Bench Get-up

Facing a bench, place your hands on the edge of the seat and extend your legs behind you in a push-up position with head, back, and feet in a straight line. Step your right leg forward in line with the right hand. Do not allow the foot to come across the body. Push through your right heel and stand up. Step back to the start position and repeat on the other leg.

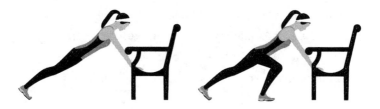

Squat Thrust Push-up

Place your hands on the seat of a bench and assume a push-up position with your head, back, and feet forming a straight line. Bend your elbows and then straighten them to raise your body. Jump towards the bench and back to the start position, keeping your hands on the bench throughout.

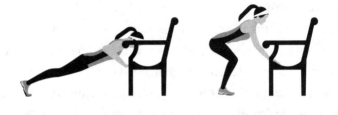

Michael's Perspective

I first started building FastStrength exercises into my regime when I came across the study "High-Intensity Circuit Training Using Body Weight" in the online version of the *American College of Sports Medicine's Health & Fitness Journal* in early 2013. As they point out at the beginning of the article, "For exercise strategies to be practical and applicable to the time-constrained client, they must be safe, effective, and efficient. As many of our clients travel frequently, the program also must be able to be performed anywhere, without special equipment." They go on to state, citing a number of studies, "that the combination of aerobic and resistance training in a high-intensity, limited-rest design can deliver numerous health benefits in much less time than traditional programs."

I travel quite a bit and have spent more evenings than I care to remember in foreign hotels. When I first read the article I was already practicing HIT. But though I was doing aerobic training I was not doing anything about body strength. So I started straightaway.

I found the exercises surprisingly easy to do, though when I am in a hotel I tend to skip the knee-high running as it seems rather unfair on anyone in the floor below who is trying to sleep.

I also discovered, on a recent trip to Australia, where I met up with some old friends from medical school, a variant called "The Park Bench Workout"—which is similar to the one proposed by Peta here.

As well as many of the exercises listed above, the Australian Park Bench Workout included one real killer, the Dip and Kick. It starts off like the tricep dip, but rapidly gets worse. You start with your hands behind you on the bench, your elbows bent at 90 degrees and your bottom a few inches off the ground. Then, instead of straightening, you have to kick out like a Russian Cossack, doing as many kicks as you can in 30 seconds.

I never really mastered this particular exercise, but on the whole FastStrength workouts have done wonders for my fitness levels. I can now do 35 push-ups in 30 seconds and 20 squats without falling over. I have rediscovered abdominal muscles that I have not seen for years. Not yet a six-pack, but getting there.

I also recently discovered, while doing push-ups at home, a pile of semi-empty pizza boxes under our bed. I'm now wondering which of the kids left them there.

What Happens When You Hit a Plateau?

As with all exercise programs, there will come a time when your body adapts to the training load that you are applying and will not respond as well as it did a few weeks previously. This is known as a fitness plateau—and we all hit them from time to time. It's at this point that you need to make tweaks to your regime, to raise your workouts to the next level so that your body begins to respond again.

This does not necessarily mean that you have to increase the duration of your session (although you can try one of the longer or shorter FastExercise workouts for variety). Progression can be achieved by increasing the intensity or speed of your "efforts," by attempting to complete more moves in an allotted time, or by shortening recovery time so that you can attempt a greater number of "bursts."

Forget the fable about the tortoise and the hare. When it comes to FastExercise it really is a case of short bursts of applied effort. In the next chapter I look at how to make FastExercise part of your daily life.

CHAPTER SEVEN

FastExercise in Practice

OVER THE YEARS I'VE CHANGED THE WAY I EXERcise to suit my lifestyle. In my teens and twenties I devoted many hours a day to improving my running times and performances. But now, as a working mum with an eight-year-old son, my day gets gobbled up with playdates, football, and rugby matches. I still crave to be outside, breathing in the fresh air of the Chilterns countryside where I live. But I no longer have the time—or desire—to do lengthy workouts. And I've found that short, sharp bursts of HIT sessions suit me perfectly.

When to Exercise

The real appeal of FastExercise is that it can slip easily into your day. Even if you are time crunched, you can always find a few minutes to devote to this kind of condensed workout. It is better, however, that you don't just "fit it in when you can." If you commit to a regular time you are more likely to keep your regime going.

So is there any evidence that exercising at any particular time of the day is more beneficial?

If you are interested in performance, then late afternoon or early evening may be a better time to work out. Researchers at Liverpool John Moores University found that when people were asked to perform the same workout at different times of the day (5 a.m., 11 a.m., 5 p.m., and 11 p.m.), they felt they were working hardest first thing—though this wasn't necessarily the case. Top swimmers have been shown to suffer a 10% drop in performance during morning training sessions.

Why? Well, your body temperature is lowest first thing in the morning. It then steadily rises by about 1 degree Celsius (33.8 degrees Fahrenheit) till it reaches a peak around midday. It stays quite high till about 7 p.m., when it starts to fall.

Being slightly more revved up with warmer muscles may contribute to an improvement in performance. It may also reduce the risk of injury. On this basis, exercising anytime between midday and 7 p.m. is good. Much later and it may disturb your sleep.

So is the afternoon best? Not necessarily. Sports scientists at Glasgow University say that, while morning exercise may feel harder for some people, it can be a great mood booster, setting you up mentally for the day. Their research, published in the journal *Appetite*,[1] found that women in an 8:15

a.m. aerobics class achieved a 50% boost to their feelings of well-being compared with 20% for those who worked out at 7:15 p.m.

There is also evidence that if you exercise before breakfast, in the fasted state, you will burn more fat.

The truth is we are all different and the best time to exercise is the time that best suits you. My optimal time is after the school run and before I settle down into my tunnel of work. I get up and get dressed in my exercise gear so that I'm ready to start exercising as soon as I get home. I've made it part of my routine so that there's less chance of my talking myself out of it.

Michael, on the other hand, splits his exercise. He does his FastStrength exercises in the morning when he gets out of bed (he finds that if he doesn't do them then he often forgets to do them at all). He gets his HIT in the early evening, by doing FastFitness training either on his bike on his way back from work or when he gets home.

What all experts agree on is that exercise at any time is better than none at all and that consistency is key to progress. American studies have shown that there are significant benefits to be gained from working out at the same time each day—interestingly, weight lifters who trained at the same time each day consistently gained more strength than those who worked out at different times—probably because they were more likely to keep at it.[2]

Are Some People Hardwired to Hate Exercise?

We've already discussed research which suggests that the amount of benefit we get from exercise is to some extent hardwired into our genes. The same may well be true of the amount of pleasure we get from exercise.

You might think that if exercise is as good for us as everyone claims we should all be primed to love it. The problem is that from an evolutionary perspective there was never any need to make exercise as enjoyable as sex or food. In the past there was no survival advantage in going for a run or doing push-ups. That would have been a waste of valuable energy at a time when calories were scarce. Our ancestors got all the "exercise" they needed from simply surviving.

Studies have shown that while some people find exercise enjoyable, for others the opposite is true; they seem to be predisposed to respond more negatively to puffing and panting than others and their mood plummets if they are forced to do it. The result? They throw in the towel early.

The beauty of FastExercise is that it is over quickly. So for those who are not blessed with a love of exercise it's a method that may be more sustainable. Certainly the HIT studies show that, though it is demanding, people prefer it to the standard, prolonged slog.

That said, most people need help if they are to stick to a new exercise regime, however short. Fortunately, just as we can train our bodies to become more efficient, so we can coax our minds to become more focused and to respond better to motivational triggers.

How to Keep Going

Starting something new is easy. It's keeping going that's hard. It helps, before you start, to be SMART about your reasons for doing an exercise regime. Thoughts like "I'd quite like to lose some weight" or "It would be nice to be a bit fitter" are not going to keep you motivated when you are tempted to lie in bed a little bit longer or take the car rather than walking. So make it:

Specific: Think about what exactly you are going to do. Specify which days and what time you are going to exercise, and give some serious thought to ensuring that it will be sustainable. If on Tuesdays you tend to work late, for example, don't put a session down for then.

Measurable: Blood markers? Waist size? VO2 max? Keep an exercise diary in which you record your baseline statistics for performance, fitness, or health, or simply the number of sessions you manage to complete in a week. Michael keeps a really fat photo of himself looking particularly unfit as a reminder.

Attainable: Goals need to be realistic and achievable. You are not going to change from an exercise-hating couch potato to a gym bunny overnight. Instead of "I will lose 10 pounds," say "I will take the stairs at work every day this week."

Rewarding: Celebrate your achievements (even just getting started). Treat yourself (though not with a muffin). Share your success with others.

Time specific: Commit to doing your chosen regime for at least three months. Once you see change you are more likely to keep going.

Strategies While Exercising

We cope with the psychological pressures of exercising in one of two ways: either we tune into our bodies and focus on what we are doing or we dissociate, think of other things, and generally try to distract ourselves.

Personally, I am what sports psychologists call an "associator"—I can run for miles without getting bored and without needing to distract myself—to "dissociate" by using music or other techniques. The good thing about HIT is that most people find that it requires such focus that there's no opportunity to get bored. Self-affirming mantras certainly help. If you need an extra kick to keep going, try shouting to yourself: "Go for it!," "Keep going," "Go, go, GO, GO!!!!," "Nearly there," "Not much longer," "I can get through this."

Pay attention to the parts of your body which are putting

in the most effort, such as your legs when pedaling or running. This will help you keep up the pace and rhythm. As you become tired, it can help to reframe or reinterpret the feeling. "This burning in my thighs is good—it means I am clearing out my arteries, burning some fat."

Maintaining your focus also means that you are more likely to hear warning signals coming from your body, telling you that you are pushing it too hard. Some days you just need to be gentle with yourself.

Eight Ways to Overcome Your Inner Couch Potato

HIT is incredibly time efficient but even so there will always be reasons not to do it. Here are some of my tips:

1. Write a pledge along the lines of "I will do a ten-minute session of HIT on the exercise bike, three times a week starting tomorrow evening when I get back from work." Pin it on the wall, schedule it into your diary, put reminders on your phone. Whatever works for you, but the more clearly you have thought it through, the more likely you are to actually do it.

2. Tell those around you what you intend to do and when. Publicly stating a goal makes you more likely to follow through.

3. Exercise with others. If you are planning on going for a jog with added HIT or perhaps you want to do a bit of FastWalking, find someone to do it with. One of the main reasons people employ trainers is to get them out of the house when they don't feel like going.

4. Join a group or a club. Set up a local group to meet regularly and exercise in the park. But don't be too ambitious as it may become another barrier to getting going. Michael says his mother has talked about joining a walking group for 30 years. She hasn't done it yet.

5. Write a list of potential excuses: can't find shoes, running clothes in the wash, I'm tired, it's cold, I'll do it tomorrow, the dog has just been sick. . . . Now address each in turn and write down the solutions. If you anticipate potential barriers, it reduces the chance of backsliding.

6. Create visual cues. Just as you are more likely to eat biscuits if they are in full view, so you are more likely to exercise if the cues are staring you in the face. Put your running shoes by the front door, move the exercise bike into the family room, find somewhere else to hang your washing other than on the cross-trainer.

7. Be aware that you have an inner voice that will tell you "this is a waste of time." Remind yourself

of your goals. Remind yourself that you will feel better afterwards. Or simply think of something else. Your inner voice is not something you have to pay attention to.

8. Your barriers will be different from mine. But they do need to be considered and also reviewed once you have started the program. Auditing your experience will make it easier to get in the habit of doing it regularly.

Food and FastExercise

As any committed exerciser or gym member will know, there's an entire industry of energy bars and sports drinks, recovery fluids and protein shakes out there. The good news? You don't need any of them to perform FastExercise. Here, instead, are a simple few dos and don'ts:

★ Don't attempt FastExercise immediately after eating. This may seem pretty obvious, but the main risk is not cramping, it's vomiting. Michael likes to do his HIT on the way home in the evening, or soon after he gets home. HIT also stops him snacking.

★ Don't load up on carbs before doing FastExercise. There is a widespread belief that carbs are needed to fuel exercise. Unless you are exercising heavily for over an hour at a time you have plenty of carbohydrates on board. Eating lots of pasta will simply make you fat.

★ Similarly, you don't need to load up on carbs *after* doing FastExercise. You may feel a bit wobbly but the whole point is to deplete your glycogen stores, so the last thing you want to do is immediately replenish them. The average person doing a HIT session three times a week does not require special "refueling."

★ As for liquids, doing FastExercise is not going to make you sweat so you are unlikely to need to drink during a session. Obviously, drink if you are thirsty. But beware of sports drinks—they are just expensive sugar. If you have been out for a long run and sweated a lot, the best way to rehydrate is with skim milk or water.

So is there anything out there that will actually help FastExercisers? Well, there are a few foods and drinks with some science behind them, as I outline below (though none of them are things I'm going to be topping myself up with on a regular basis):

Beetroot juice: Beetroot juice is rich in nitrates which increases the levels of nitric oxide in the body. Nitric oxide affects a range of things, including blood flow and cell signaling. Scientists at the University of Exeter found that volunteers who drank 500 milliliters (16.9 ounces) of beetroot juice a day for a week could keep going for longer before getting tired. We may yet see beetroot-loaded athletes at the next Olympics. Beetroot juice is an acquired taste.

Cherry juice: Studies at Northumbria University showed that drinking tart cherry juice twice a day for five days before a marathon resulted in quicker recovery and less muscle pain after the event. The phytochemicals, especially anthocyanins, found in sour Montmorency cherries in particular have anti-inflammatory and antioxidating properties which seem to aid recovery. However, the benefits are clear only in endurance runners. For the rest of us it's just calories.

Bicarbonate of soda: Another unlikely drink that might benefit top athletes but which is unlikely to help the rest of us is bicarbonate of soda. In a small study some swimmers who took baking soda an hour before a 200-meter event shaved a second or so off their usual performances. If you are keen, then about 20 grams (4 teaspoons) should do it, in a little water, before exercise and on an empty stomach. Potential soda dopers should be warned that it tastes vile and can cause upset stomachs.

Ginger: Ginger root is known to have anti-inflammatory and pain-relieving effects and a randomized controlled study done at the University of Georgia[3] showed that daily ginger consumption reduces muscle pain after exercise. Subjects were asked to take ginger capsules or a placebo for eleven consecutive days and then to perform a series of tough exercises on the eighth day. Ginger supplementation reduced exercise-induced pain by 25%. It's certainly better than taking ibuprofen.

Kids and HIT

We can learn a lot from children. If you have ever spent time in a primary school playground or at a play park, you will have witnessed the most unadulterated display of HIT-style exercise in action. For children of ten and under, HIT comes naturally.

I have watched my own eight-year-old son sprint and recover his way around a walk with our border collie, perfectly unaware that he is performing the kind of exercise that is taking the scientific world by storm. At that age their bodies are physiologically primed to move fast in short bursts. Young aerobic systems switch on more quickly than those of adults, producing the energy needed for movement, regardless of its intensity. And children's short attention spans mean they are perfectly suited to the stop-start style of FastExercise.

But this doesn't mean they should be performing HIT workouts such as those outlined in this book. Structured exercise at a young age should be limited to the occasional football or netball game. Children need to engage in activity freely and uninhibitedly, without pressure and without a stopwatch—indeed, without realizing they are doing it at all.

Kids are a good example to us all. Not only are they natural FastExercisers, they tend to move about and fidget a lot. And this, as Michael will outline in the next chapter, is key. While HIT is all well and good, it's not enough on its own. The ideal is to combine it with being generally more active.

CHAPTER EIGHT

Michael's Guide to Keeping Active

YOU MIGHT WANT TO READ THIS SECTION OF THE book while standing up. Or perhaps while strolling around. Remember that the hunter-gatherer approach, which we encountered in Chapter 5, involves much more than simply doing short bursts of intense exercise. It also means increasing the amount of activity that you build into your everyday life. It is the combination of the two that will have a dramatic effect on your health, fitness, weight, and well-being.

All of us have benefited from the technological advances that have occurred in our lifetimes. Our homes are packed full of labor-saving devices. We love our smart phones, email, and TVs. But technology also has a lot to answer for. It has made us unbelievably slothful.

Do you know—though why would you—what the average waist-size of a middle-aged woman was in the 1950s?

An impressively svelte 28 inches. And now it's 34 inches. That 6-inch expansion—6 inches of unrequired and unloved fat—is partly due to the fact that modern women do not burn anything like as many calories doing housework as their grandmothers did. This is not because women have become more slovenly or, I might add, because men have stepped up to the mark and are doing more around the house—no, men are pretty much as idle around the house as they were a generation ago. The problem is those lovely labor-saving devices.

Sixty years ago a woman could comfortably burn her way through 1,000 calories a day just by doing the chores—washing, mopping, and cleaning. These days we let machines take the strain. Very few people would wish to wind back the clock, but somehow we have to find a way to increase the calorie consumption in our lives.

Ditch the Chair

Guess how many hours a day you spend sitting? Less than 8? More than 10? Some experts claim that many of us spend up to 12 hours a day sitting on our well-padded bottoms looking at computers or watching television. If you throw in the 8 hours we spend sleeping, then that adds up to a remarkable 20 hours a day being sedentary. Ouch.

The trouble is that we all kid ourselves about how much we move. To find out just how much, or little, I move in an average day I met up with the incredibly enthusiastic and hyperactive Jim Levine. Jim, who is a professor of medicine at the Mayo Clinic in the United States, has had a lifelong passion for studying movement. When he was young he would measure the average speed that slugs and snails traveled around in his garden. He is still studying the slothful and sluggardly, but these days he has more sophisticated equipment and his subjects are larger. Much larger.

According to Jim, an obesity specialist, the secret of a long and healthy life lies in improving what he calls your NEAT, your Non-Exercise Activity Thermogenesis. As Jim explained, NEAT is about the calories we burn through ordinary everyday living—getting up in the morning, going to bed at night, and all the movements you do while you're sleeping.

To keep the fuels moving through our systems we need to be moving every half an hour or so. And yet, as Jim told me, many of us now regularly spend twelve hours a day in a chair. It is an extraordinary statistic.

"Sedentariness alone appears to be a killer," he said. "Bound to the chair, chained to the chair . . . it's hurting our bodies, it's literally killing millions. Who'd have ever thought that the chair could kill?"

The trouble is that being seated doesn't just burn a bare minimum of calories—sinister things happen when we are inactive for too long. Prolonged sitting has been linked to a sharp reduction in the activity of an important enzyme called lipoprotein lipase which breaks down blood fats and makes them available as a fuel to the muscles. This reduction in enzyme activity leads to raised levels of triglycerides and fats in the blood, increasing the risk of heart disease. Extended sitting has also been shown to cause sharp spikes in blood sugar levels after meals, creating the perfect setting for type 2 diabetes.

Now, I think of myself as quite active, and I found it hard to believe that I was as slothful as Jim suggested. Twelve hours a day sitting down? I challenged him to prove it. At which point he pulled out of his smart leather briefcase a pair of the most extraordinary underpants I have ever seen.

"This," Jim explained, "is NEAT underwear, known more colloquially as fidget pants."

The pants are fitted with multiple sensors and accelerometers designed to detect—and to store on a microprocessor—every movement made by the wearer. "So if you wear these for a day," Jim continued, "we can see everything you were doing 20 times a second, night and day."

Two weeks later, we met up again to get the results, standing up of course. Jim's reaction was not encouraging. "Oh dear, oh dear, oh dear!" he said. Apparently my fidget pants had revealed that in an average day there was not a lot of fidgeting going on at all. There was move, stop, move, stop, but most of it was stop. In fact, Jim's pants suggested I spent at least eleven hours a day sitting down, sometimes for several hours at a time. During long meetings I became positively comatose.

This was sobering. I was aware that I spent quite a lot of time sitting and thinking, but certainly not that much. So I decided to see what would happen if I made a deliberate attempt to keep on my feet more.

I put the magic pants back on and for the next 24 hours I made a concerted effort to keep on the move, without actually exercising. I found it impossible to avoid my desk completely, but I did avoid the lift and took every opportunity to get up and just stroll around a bit, brainstorming with colleagues while on the move.

When I returned a while later, pants in hand, Jim was extremely encouraging. "Congratulations," he said, "you doubled your amount of NEAT. I mean, we're talking 500 extra calories burned in one day through some simple changes. And how much sweat did you drip doing this? I'm betting none. . . ."

Keeping on the move isn't just a good way of burning calories. It also has a big impact on your health. In a recent study from Australia[1] researchers gathered 70 healthy adults and asked them to do a series of experiments which involved an awful lot of sitting.

In the first part of the experiment they were asked to sit for nine hours straight. Every few hours they were asked to knock back a meal replacement drink. Soon after having their delicious drink they had their blood glucose levels and insulin levels measured.

Then they did it all over again, exactly the same, except this time they were asked to walk around at a brisk pace for half an hour before they did a nine-hour sitting stint.

They were then asked to do it one final time, except on this occasion they had to get up and walk around for exactly 1 minute and 40 seconds every 30 minutes.

On analyzing the data, the researchers discovered that

when the volunteers got up and walked every half hour their bodies were much better at coping with the meal replacement drinks. There wasn't the same surge in either glucose or insulin that they saw when the volunteers just sat. In fact, their blood glucose levels went down by 39%, while their insulin levels also fell by an impressive 26%.

What this and other studies clearly show is that we need to move more. Short bursts of activity can be as effective as much longer periods of continuous activity at improving sugar and fat levels.

So if you do spend a lot of your work life sitting down, find an excuse to get up and move—every 30 minutes.

Where Are the Stairs?

There are many ways in which modern society conspires to keep us burning as few calories as possible, the most obvious example being the car. But one of my particular beefs is stairs. Why are buildings designed so that the stairs are so incredibly hard to find and use? I try to take the stairs as often as I can, but all too frequently they are hidden somewhere inaccessible. And they're usually uninviting too.

Escalators and walkways are just as bad. As soon as people step on an escalator they freeze, blocking the way for everyone else. The really depressing thing is that despite what we know about the benefits of keeping moving, modern architectural design seems to be taking us in the opposite direction.

When sports scientists at Loughborough University

looked at the availability of stairs in newly built shopping centers, airports, and other public places, they found there were pitifully few. Architects design new buildings with escalators and lifts to comply with access requirements—in which the stairs are not there to be used, except in a fire evacuation.

Yet as Professor Gregory Heath, from the School of Public Health at the University of Tennessee, has repeatedly pointed out, one of the best ways to make people more active is to provide motivational signs directing them to use the stairs instead of the lifts. It only works, of course, if they can find them.

Our advice? Find the stairs, and use them whenever you can. They are not just for HIT. You can also use them to move from floor to floor.

10,000 Steps

The easiest way to get more active is to walk. As I mentioned earlier, a typical hunter-gatherer walks 6–10 kilometers (3.7–6.2 miles) a day. That comes to roughly 10,000 steps, the currently recommended level of activity that we should all be aiming at. Many of us don't get close.

In *The Step Diet*,[2] the authors quote a Harris poll in which 1,000 Americans were asked to wear step counters (pedometers) for two days. They found that people who were overweight walked nearly 2,000 fewer steps a day than those who were slimmer and that half of all women over 50 didn't reach even half the recommended levels (men did slightly better).

Walking will only burn modest numbers of calories, but if you do it enough and on a regular basis it all adds up. Walking also has other, more subtle benefits—not the least of which is that, unlike jogging, it does not seem to lead to compensatory eating.

To discover just how much difference walking can make I took part in an unusual experiment organized by Dr. Jason Gill of Glasgow University.

We met on a cold winter's morning in a Scottish café where Jason suggested I eat a large breakfast. Bacon, eggs, sausages, and bread, all fried in butter and oil.

"The amount of fat in that breakfast," he told me, "is similar to the amount of fat people eat during the course of a day. The fat's going to go into your gut, and then into your bloodstream, where it's going to cause a number of changes to your metabolism, and all these things are going to increase the risk of fatty deposits forming on the walls of your blood vessels."

I paused, fork halfway to my mouth, to digest this thought. "If you think that sounds bad," he added helpfully, "wait till you see it."

Four hours after my breakfast Jason took a sample of my blood, which he then spun in a high-speed centrifuge to separate the various elements. "That's the fat from the food that you've eaten, right there," he said, pointing to a creamy, milky fluid sitting at the top of the test tube. "That's the stuff that's been circulating round your body for the last couple of hours. If we compare this with a blood sample taken before you ate breakfast you can see that eating all that fried food has doubled the amount of fat in your bloodstream."

Slightly shaken, I headed off for a walk. Jason assured me that walking even a few miles would make a measurable difference.

The next morning I went back to the same café to complete part two of the experiment. I ate exactly the same meal. Four hours after eating, Jason again took a sample of my blood and after much spinning and separating presented me with the results.

"You can see," he said, "that there's substantially less fat in the sample today than there was yesterday. Today you've got about a third less fat going round your bloodstream, a third less fat interacting with the walls of your blood vessels."

The walking I had done the previous afternoon had switched on genes that make an enzyme called lipoprotein lipase, and it was this enzyme that produced the striking 33% fall in the amount of circulating fat. I was impressed and immediately went out and bought a pedometer.

These days whenever I'm tempted to drive a short distance that I could easily walk I remember Jason's test tubes.

High-Intensity Interval Walking—FastWalking

Walking is good, but FastWalking is better. Like other forms of FastExercise activity, FastWalking involves alternating walking fast with walking slow.

In a recent study published in *Diabetes Care*,[3] 24 volunteers with type 2 diabetes were asked to walk for an hour a day, five days a week. Twelve of them were asked to walk at a constant speed, the other twelve alternated three minutes of brisk walking with three minutes of gentle walking. The volunteers all wore accelerometers and heart-rate monitors to ensure that both groups were doing the same amount of work, burning the same number of calories.

At the end of the four-month trial they found that the volunteers who had done FastWalking had improved their VO2 max by 16%, lost fat, and improved their blood glucose control. The changes were far greater than in those who had walked at a constant speed.

In another study from Japan[4] involving 248 men and women in which researchers compared three minutes' fast-slow walking with continuous speed walking, they again saw much greater improvements in the FastWalking group. In this study the volunteers did five bursts of FastWalking a day, four days a week.

For suggestions on how to do a FastWalking workout see pages 311–312.

12 Easy Ways to Introduce More Activity into Our Lives

The following suggestions come mainly from the Mayo Clinic, where Professor Jim Levine is based.

1. Stand while talking on the phone. You'll burn calories and sound more assertive.

2. If you work at a desk for long periods you might consider buying a standing desk. This is a desk at which, as the name implies, you stand. Winston Churchill apparently wrote some of his famous speeches while working at one.

3. If you have to sit, try using a chair with no back, or even one of those giant sit-on balls. This strengthens core muscles and prevents slumping (and therefore backache).

4. Go and see a colleague instead of sending an email.

5. Walk laps with the other members of a meeting rather than gather in a conference room.

6. Drink lots of water. This not only keeps you hydrated but it also increases the need for bathroom breaks, which means in turn more short, brisk walks.

7. Rather than taking a break with a coffee or a snack, take a stroll or go up and down the stairs.

8. If you normally take a bus or train to work, get off at an earlier stop than usual and walk the rest of the way.

9. If you drive to work, park at the far end of the car park.

10. Keep resistance bands—stretchy cords or tubes that offer resistance when you pull on them—or small hand weights near your desk. Do arm curls between meetings or tasks.

11. Organize a lunchtime walking group. You might be surrounded by people who are just dying to lace up their trainers. Enjoy the camaraderie, and offer encouragement to one another when you feel like backsliding.

12. If you're stuck in an airport, don't sit down. Grab your bags and go look around the shops.

In Summary . . .

We cannot stress enough that FastExercise will be fully effective only if you lead an otherwise active life. One of the dispiriting things that happen as we get older is that we tend, almost imperceptibly, to put on weight. The pounds creep up on us—generally at a rate of 2–3 pounds (1–1.5 kilograms) a year—barely noticeable at first, but eventually forcing us up a whole size in clothes. Much of this gain is down to general inactivity.

On average, thin people stand for around two hours longer every day than those who carry more weight. Simply by standing more, pacing around a bit more, taking the stairs, and walking when you can, you should burn through at least an extra 350 calories a day. Over a year this adds up to the calorie equivalent of running about 1,000 miles.

CHAPTER NINE

Before You Go . . .

A S WE'VE SEEN, THE SCIENCE OF EXERCISE IS MOV-ing fast. HIT—ultrashort bursts of intense activity—has been shown to be an extremely time-efficient way to improve fitness and health, particularly when combined (as in the hunter-gatherer approach) with increased levels of general activity; and its use is gradually extending, from athletes and the young and healthy to those who are older and less fit.

As with all forms of exercise it's important not to overdo or rush into HIT; but I find it encouraging (and surprising) that so far its safety and effectiveness have stood up to being tested in people who are most at risk, those with a history of heart disease and stroke.

The joy of FastExercise, of course, is that the exertion is short-lived: it is the perfect workout for the time-starved generation. It can fit unobtrusively into your day— so much so that, if you stick with it, it soon becomes habitual.

There are few miracles in this world, and this book is not offering you a magic wand. What we recommend is rather a shift in your perception, so that you come to see exercise not as an unwelcome chore to be got over and done with— yet another thing on your To Do list, to be slotted in at the end of a hard week—but instead as a small, but key part of your daily life, an activity almost as instinctual as getting up in the morning and brushing your teeth. In this way, FastExercise should become sustainable and, dare I say it, even enjoyable.

And this is the case whether you are an aerobic high responder who already enjoys doing lots of exercise, like Peta, or a low responder who does not, like me.

For high responders, HIT offers a rapid, high-impact regime that can be added to existing workouts to maximize their effectiveness. For the sloths among us, HIT is a joy because it liberates us from the hell of slogging round the running track or going to the gym (which, let's be honest, we are never going to do), while still delivering many of the other wonders of exercise, including increased fat burning. Though be aware that without watching your calories no exercise regime will ever lead to long-term weight loss.

So far studies on HIT have largely been confined to athletes, hospitals, and the laboratory. Plans are under way to study its effectiveness in real-life settings, particularly in the workplace. I await the results of those studies with interest.

Another area of research that this book has tried to highlight is the danger of the chair. The chair is not simply a useful bit of furniture, it is a killer. Instead of spending hours at a time hunched over our computers or televisions, allowing the sugar and fat from our last meal to clog up our arteries, we need to recognize the importance of intermittent movement, to find reasons to get up from our chairs and go for a short stroll or even just have a brief stretch at least once every half hour.

The fact that we are becoming increasingly sedentary, with all the problems that this leads to (increased risk of diabetes, heart disease, dementia, to name but a few), is surely evidence that public exhortations and health messages are not enough. We need help to overcome our inner sloth. And some of this has to come from above. There are examples, though not nearly enough, of cities where politicians, architects, planners, and employers have come together to make changes to the physical environment—changes that encourage us to burn calories rather than simply add them to our burgeoning bellies. We need more city centers where it is safe to cycle and where cars are banned or severely limited; buildings with stairs that are visible, attractive, and inviting to use; escalators that invite us to walk rather than stay rooted to the spot.

We were born to move. Some of us more reluctantly than others. So let's find ways to do it more. Fast.

Ways to Measure the Impact of Exercise

You can do the following calculations yourself or visit our website, fast-exercises.com, where you can obtain more information, get the calculations done automatically, and join a forum to discuss all things exercise-related.

The Importance of Heart Rate

Your resting heart rate is itself a powerful predictor of future health. According to a study of 11,000 people published in the *Lancet* (September 2008), those with heart rates above 70 beats per minute are at greater risk of heart attack and hospital admission. With regular exercise you should see your resting heart rate fall.

Top athletes can have a resting pulse as low as 40 beats per minute. Mine is around 64 beats per minute.

Your resting heart rate is easy to find. Turn your hand so your palm is facing you. Use your index and middle finger from your other hand to measure it at the wrist, just below the thumb. Measure it when you are sitting down and relaxed, preferably first thing in the morning.

Heart Rate Max (HR Max)

Some of the exercises in this book talk about pushing yourself to 80% or 90% of your maximum heart rate. So how do you measure that? The most direct way is to run or cycle as fast as you can against resistance for about three minutes, rest for a couple of minutes, then try pushing yourself as hard as possible for another couple of minutes. Your heart rate will probably peak at some point during the second burst. This should not be attempted if you have any doubts about your fitness.

When I did it, the highest I could get my heart rate to was 164, so my HR max is 164.

If you prefer something less stressful, the safest way to get an estimate of your HR max is by using one of the formulas for calculating it, of which the best known is 220 minus your age for men and 226 minus your age for women. It is simple, but out of date, and a more reliable version for both sexes is HR max = 205.8—(0.685 x age).

On this basis my HR max is 167, which is close to what I found in practice.

Knowing your HR max will help you calculate how hard to push yourself when you are doing some of the HIT exercises in the book, though you will probably also need a heart-rate monitor as stopping to measure your heart rate while you are exercising is tricky.

HR max will also help you calculate your VO2 max.

VO2 Max

VO2 max is a measure of aerobic fitness, one of the most important predictors of future health. The most reliable way to find your VO2 max is to have it done in a lab or a gym that has suitable facilities. But if you don't have access to a lab there are other ways to estimate your aerobic fitness.

The simplest is the Uth–Sørensen–Overgaard–Pedersen estimation:

VO2 max = 15.3 x HR max/HR rest

Since my HR max is 164 and my resting heart rate is 64, according to this formula my VO2 max = 15.3 x 164/64 = 39.2 mL/(kg.min).

This is reasonably close to the result I got when my VO2 max was tested in the lab, which was 37 mL/(kg.min). (Just to put that in perspective: Peta's VO2 max is a whopping 53 mL/(kg.min), which is very high for a woman, let alone one of her age. Actually, by my standards, it's high for a man too.)

Once you have estimated your VO2 max use the charts on the facing page to see how well you are doing. For my age I am rated "good."

Unless you are an aerobic nonresponder you should see improvements in your VO2 max after six weeks of following a FastExercise regime.

Before You Go . . .

WOMEN							
AGE (YEARS)	VERY POOR	POOR	FAIR	AVERAGE	GOOD	VERY GOOD	EXCELLENT
20–24	<27	27–31	32–36	37–41	42–46	47–51	>51
25–29	<26	26–30	31–35	36–40	41–44	45–49	>49
30–34	<25	25–29	30–33	34–37	38–42	43–46	>46
35–39	<24	24–27	28–31	32–35	36–40	41–44	>44
40–44	<22	22–25	26–29	30–33	34–37	38–41	>41
45–49	<21	21–23	24–27	28–31	32–35	36–38	>38
50–54	<19	19–22	23–25	26–29	30–32	33–36	>36
55–59	<18	18–20	21–23	24–27	28–30	31–33	>33
60–65	<16	16–18	19–21	22–24	25–27	28–30	>30

MEN							
AGE (YEARS)	VERY POOR	POOR	FAIR	AVERAGE	GOOD	VERY GOOD	EXCELLENT
20–24	<32	32–37	38–43	44–50	51–56	57–62	>62
25–29	<31	31–35	36–42	43–48	49–53	54–59	>59
30–34	<29	29–34	35–40	41–45	46–51	52–56	>56
35–39	<28	28–32	33–38	39–43	44–48	49–54	>54
40–44	<26	26–31	32–35	36–41	42–46	47–51	>51
45–49	<25	25–29	30–34	35–39	40–43	44–48	>48
50–54	<24	24–27	28–32	33–36	37–41	42–46	>46
55–59	<22	22–26	27–30	31–34	35–39	40–43	>43
60–65	<21	21–24	25–28	29–32	33–36	37–40	>40

The Rockport One Mile Walk Test

This is a better way of estimating VO2 max. You walk a mile as briskly as you can, then measure your heart rate at the end.

The formula:

VO2 max = 132.853 – (0.0769 × weight) – (0.3877 × age) + (6.315 × gender) – (3.2649 × time) – (0.1565 × heart rate)

1. You enter your weight in pounds.

2. Gender male = 1 and female = 0.

3. You measure the time you take to walk the mile in minutes and seconds.

I'm 164 pounds, 56 years old, male. I did the walk in 14 minutes and 30 seconds (14.5 minutes) and my heart rate was 120 beats per minute at the end:

VO2 max = 132.853 – (0.0769 × 164) – (0.3877 × 56) + (6.315 × 1) – (3.2649 × 14.5) – (0.1565 × 120) = 132.9 – 12.6 – 21.7 + 6.3 – 47.3 – 18.8 = 38.7

Alternative Ways of Assessing Aerobic Fitness

The Cooper Run

Another long-standing test was devised for the United States Air Force by physiologist Kenneth Cooper and first published in the *Journal of the American Medical Association* back in 1968. It is still widely used by athletes and football teams. In its original form the test requires you to run as far as you can in twelve minutes on a 400-meter athletics track (so that distance can be measured accurately to the nearest 10 meters). Your aerobic fitness can then be estimated from the following table:

COOPER TEST (20–50+)						
		VERY GOOD	GOOD	AVERAGE	BAD	VERY BAD
20–29	M	2800+ m	2400–2800 m	2200–2399 m	1600–2199 m	1600– m
	F	2700+ m	2200–2700 m	1800–2199 m	1500–1799 m	1500– m
30–39	M	2700+ m	2300–2700 m	1900–2299 m	1500–1899 m	1500– m
	F	2500+ m	2000–2500 m	1700–1999 m	1400–1699 m	1400– m
40–49	M	2500+ m	2100–2500 m	1700–2099 m	1400–1699 m	1400– m
	F	2300+ m	1900–2300 m	1500–1899 m	1200–1499 m	1200– m

continued on next page

| 50+ | M | 2400+ m | 2000–2400 m | 1600–1999 m | 1300–1599 m | 1300– m |
| | F | 2200+ m | 1700–2200 m | 1400–1699 m | 1100–1399 m | 1100– m |

COOPER TEST (EXPERIENCED ATHLETES)					
		VERY GOOD	GOOD	AVERAGE	BAD	VERY BAD
	M	3700+ m	3400–3700 m	3100–3399 m	2800–3099 m	2800– m
	F	2200+ m	2700–3000 m	2400–2699 m	2100–2399 m	2100– m

Oral Glucose Tolerance Test

One of the most important things that regular exercise does is help your body cope with high levels of blood glucose after a meal.

Persistently elevated blood sugar, even if it isn't in the diabetic range, is a bad sign. Unless it is removed, excess glucose binds to body proteins (a process called glycation), damaging arteries and nerves. This, in turn, can lead to blindness, impotence, dementia, and heart disease.

The oral glucose tolerance test is an important measure of your metabolic fitness, how well and how quickly your body deals with glucose. It is a test that is best done by your doctor but it can also be done at home—though this should not be attempted at home if you are a Type 1 or Type 2 diabetic, if you suffer from needle phobia, or have any reason to believe you will respond badly to a significant sugar hit.

The test consists of consuming 75 grams (2.6 ounces) of

fast-acting carbohydates, either as a drink or as food, on an empty stomach, then measuring the effects that has on your blood glucose levels.

If you are doing it at home, then first you have to buy a simple blood glucose monitoring kit from your pharmacist or online.

- You need to fast overnight for a minimum of ten hours (only water permitted).

- You then dissolve 75 grams (2.6 ounces) of glucose in 300 milliliters (10 ounces) of water. You can buy glucose from a pharmacist or online. Ordinary table sugar, sucrose, is made up of glucose and fructose, so it is not the same. It needs to be drunk within a couple of minutes.

- Alternatively you can drink 380 milliliters (12.8 ounces) of Lucozade Original.

- If you prefer, 8 ounces (227 grams) of boiled potato will deliver roughly the same level of carbohydrates. Nothing else to be eaten with it, though.

- The main thing is be consistent if you decide to repeat the test months later.

Once you've drunk the glucose or eaten the potato, record the time. At the end of one hour, and then again at two hours, prick your finger and measure your blood glucose levels, recording the results.

How to Interpret the Results

Too high? By the end of two hours your glucose levels should have fallen below 7.4 mmol/L (120 mg/dl). If that hasn't happened then you may be diabetic or have impaired glucose tolerance. See your doctor, who will probably repeat the tests in a more controlled setting.

Too low? If your blood sugar goes high after one hour but then drops below 3.9 mmol/L (70 mg/dl) at two hours you may have "reactive hypoglycemia." After drinking the glucose or eating the carbs your blood sugar went up, so your pancreas pumped out insulin to bring it down. But it was too much so you ended up with low blood sugar. The symptoms are wide-ranging but may include fatigue and dizziness. Again, see your doctor.

If your blood glucose is elevated above 6.1 mmol/L (110 mg/dL), then do keep an eye on it. Six weeks of FastExercise should improve your body's ability to cope with glucose. Let us know, via the website, how you get on.

Muscular Fitness

Doing regular FastStrength exercises should, depending on your genes, make you stronger. One way of assessing this is by the number of push-ups you can do in one minute. If you are unfit (or a woman) you may want to start with a modified push-up, kneeling down and then pushing yourself up.

The following chart is based on research done—like the

aerobic fitness test, on page 360—at the Cooper Institute for Aerobics Research in Dallas, Texas, where they have collected data on over 100,000 people. As I mentioned, Kenneth Cooper was an air force doctor who carried out some of the first extensive research on aerobic exercise and wrote a bestseller, *Aerobics,* in 1968. Among other groups, the Cooper Institute works with the military and the police. Apparently American policemen tend to be overweight, aerobically unfit, but stronger than the average person.

MEN: FULL BODY PUSH-UPS					
AGE	**20–29**	**30–39**	**40–49**	**50–59**	**60+**
Superior	62	52	40	39	28
Excellent	47	39	35	30	23
Good	37	30	24	19	18
Fair	29	24	18	13	10
Poor	22	17	11	9	6
Very poor	13	9	5	3	2

WOMEN: MODIFIED PUSH-UPS					
AGE	**20–29**	**30–39**	**40–49**	**50–59**	**60+**
Superior	45	39	33	28	20
Excellent	36	31	24	21	15
Good	30	24	18	17	12
Fair	23	19	13	12	5
Poor	11	7	6	6	2
Very poor	9	4	1	0	0

WOMEN: FULL PUSH-UPS			
AGE	20–29	30–39	40–49
Superior	42	39	20
Excellent	28	23	15
Good	21	15	13
Fair	15	11	9
Poor	10	8	6
Very poor	3	1	0

I started out in the "good" range, able to do 20 push-ups in a minute. After a couple of months doing high-intensity circuit training, I am now able to do 40 in a minute, which I'm pleased to say pushes me into "superior."

Peta, being a runner, has not focused on strength and she is not keen on push-ups. She tells me she can manage about 20 modified push-ups in a minute. "Good."

Get on the Scales

An obvious thing you will want to do before embarking on this adventure is to weigh yourself. Initially, it is best to do this at the same time every day. First thing in the morning is, as I'm sure you know, when you will be at your lightest.

Ideally, you should get a weighing machine that measures body-fat percentage as well as weight, since what you really want to see is your body-fat levels fall and muscle rise. The cheaper machines are not fantastically reliable;

they tend to underestimate the true figure, giving you a false sense of security. What they are quite good at doing, however, is measuring change. In other words, they might tell you when you start that you are 30% body fat when the true figure is closer to 33%. But they should be able to tell you when that number begins to fall.

Body Fat

Body fat is measured as a percentage of total weight. The machines you can buy do this by a system called impedence. They generate a small electric current that runs through your body and measures the resistance to it. The estimation is based on the fact that muscle and other tissues are better conductors of electricity than fat.

The only way to get a truly accurate figure is with a machine called a DXA (formerly DEXA) scanner. It stands for "Dual Energy X-ray Absorptiometry." It is expensive and for most people unnecessary. Your body mass index (BMI) will tell you if you are overweight. Women tend to have more body fat than men. A man with body fat of more than 25% would be considered overweight. For a woman it would be 30%.

Calculate Your BMI

To calculate your BMI, go to a website such as http://www
.nhs.uk/Tools/Pages/Healthyweightcalculator.aspx. This will
not only do the calculation, but also tell you what it means.
One criticism of BMI is that someone who has a lot of muscle could get a high BMI score. This is not an issue for most
of us, sadly.

Measure Your Stomach

BMI is useful but it may not be the best predictor of future
health. In a study of over 45,000 women followed for sixteen years, it was the waist-to-height ratio that proved a
superior predictor of who would develop heart disease.

The reason the waist matters so much is because the
worst sort of fat is visceral fat, which collects inside the abdomen. Most people think that fat is fat and all fat is equal.
Recently it has become clear that this is not true. Subcutaneous fat, the sort of fat you get on your arms, legs, and buttocks, is unsightly but has relatively little impact on health.
The visceral fat coats and infiltrates your internal organs like
your liver and your pancreas. It causes inflammation and
puts you at much higher risk of diabetes.

You would imagine that if you had lots of visceral fat you
would have to look fat, but this is not the case. I only discovered that I was a TOFI (Thin on the Outside, Fat Inside)

when I went for an MRI scan as part of a documentary. I didn't look overweight but the scan revealed that in fact I had many liters of internal fat. Around 25% of people who have a normal BMI will have worrying levels of visceral fat, without knowing it. Although it is not ideal, if you can't afford an MRI or a DXA scan, the simplest and cheapest test is a tape measure.

Male or female, your waist should be less than half your height. Most people underestimate their waist size by about two inches because they rely on trouser size. Instead, measure your waist by putting the tape measure around your belly button. Be honest. A definition of optimism is someone who steps on the scales while holding their breath. You are fooling no one.

Calories Burned Doing Different Activities

This chart is here more for general interest than anything else. I find that when I am tempted to eat a calorie-laden muffin (and I am, regularly), then I just think about how much activity I will have to do to burn off those calories. These figures are gross. To get net calories burned you have to subtract your basal metabolic rate (BMR), the calories that you would have burned sitting down doing nothing. Your BMR depends on your age, weight, sex, and height. Mine is around 67 calories per hour.

ACTIVITY, EXERCISE, OR SPORT (1 HOUR)	130 lbs	155 lbs	180 lbs	205 lbs
Walking the dog	177	211	245	279
Squash	708	844	981	1117
Ballroom dancing, slow	177	211	245	279
Ballroom dancing, fast	325	387	449	512
Running up stairs	885	1056	1226	1396
Archery	207	246	286	326
Badminton	266	317	368	419
Basketball	354	422	490	558
Billiards	148	176	204	233
Bowling	177	211	245	279
Cricket (batting, bowling)	295	352	409	465
Croquet	148	176	204	233
Darts	148	176	204	233
Fencing	354	422	490	558
Frisbee playing	177	211	245	279
Golf, general	266	317	368	419
Riding a horse	236	281	327	372
Horse grooming, vigorous	354	422	490	558
Martial arts, judo, karate, kick-boxing	590	704	817	931
Juggling	236	281	327	372
Rock-climbing	649	774	899	1024
Jumping rope	590	704	817	931
Skateboarding	295	352	409	465
Roller-skating	413	493	572	651
Rollerblading	708	844	981	1117
Skydiving	177	211	245	279
Football, competitive	590	704	817	931

ACTIVITY, EXERCISE, OR SPORT (1 HOUR)	130 lbs	155 lbs	180 lbs	205 lbs
Football, noncompetitive	413	493	572	651
Table tennis, Ping Pong	236	281	327	372
Tai chi	236	281	327	372
Tennis, doubles	354	422	490	558
Tennis, singles	472	563	654	745
Trampoline	207	246	286	326
Volleyball, beach	472	563	654	745
Backpacking, Hiking	413	493	572	651
Carrying a child, level ground	207	246	286	326
Carrying a child, up stairs	295	352	409	465
Carrying 16 to 24 lbs, up stairs	354	422	490	558
Carrying 25 to 49 lbs, up stairs	472	563	654	745
Standing, chatting	165	197	229	261
Walking/running, playing with children, moderate	236	281	327	372
Loading, unloading car	177	211	245	279
Climbing hills, carrying up to 9 lbs	413	493	572	651
Climbing hills, carrying 10 to 20 lbs	443	528	613	698
Climbing hills, carrying 21 to 42 lbs	472	563	654	745
Climbing hills, carrying over 42 lbs	531	633	735	838
Walking down stairs	177	211	245	279
Bird-watching	148	176	204	233
Marching, rapidly, military	384	457	531	605
Children's games like hopscotch	295	352	409	465
Pushing a stroller or walking with children	148	176	204	233
Pushing a wheelchair	236	281	327	372
Walking using crutches	295	352	409	465
Walking 2.0 mph, slow	148	176	204	233

ACTIVITY, EXERCISE, OR SPORT (1 HOUR)	130 lbs	155 lbs	180 lbs	205 lbs
Walking 3.0 mph, moderate	195	232	270	307
Walking 3.5 mph, uphill	354	422	490	558
Walking 4.0 mph, brisk	295	352	409	465
Walking 5.0 mph	472	563	654	745
Boating, powerboat, speedboat	148	176	204	233
Crew, sculling, rowing, competition	708	844	981	1117
Kayaking	295	352	409	465
Skiing, waterskiing	354	422	490	558
Snorkeling	295	352	409	465
Surfing	177	211	245	279
White-water rafting, kayaking, canoeing	295	352	409	465
Treading water, vigorous	590	704	817	931
Treading water, moderate	236	281	327	372
Water aerobics	236	281	327	372
Water polo	590	704	817	931
Water volleyball	177	211	245	279
Diving, springboard or platform	177	211	245	279
Ice-skating, average speed	413	493	572	651
Sledding, tobogganing	413	493	572	651
Snowmobiling	207	246	286	326
General housework	207	246	286	326
Cleaning gutters	295	352	409	465
Painting	266	317	368	419
Sitting, playing with animals	148	176	204	233
Walking/running, playing with animals	236	281	327	372
Mowing lawn, walking, power mower	325	387	449	512
Mowing lawn, riding mower	148	176	204	233

ACTIVITY, EXERCISE, OR SPORT (1 HOUR)	130 lbs	155 lbs	180 lbs	205 lbs
Shoveling snow by hand	354	422	490	558
Raking lawn	254	303	351	400
Gardening, general	236	281	327	372
Watering lawn or garden	89	106	123	140
Carpentry, general	207	246	286	326
Carrying heavy loads	472	563	654	745
Taking out the trash	177	211	245	279
Teaching physical education, exercise class	236	281	327	372
Teaching and participating in exercise class	384	457	531	605

FastFitness

Depending on your fitness level, there are several workouts you can perform, all described on pages 293–300. These should be done 2–3 times a week, and you can choose among the exercises below:

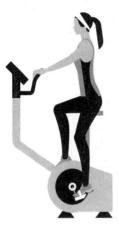

Cycling: Sprint from 20 seconds to four minutes depending on which FastFitness session you choose.

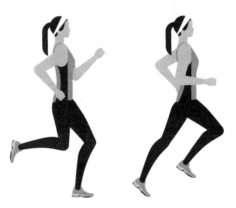

Running: Start by running flat-out up a hill for 10 seconds. Slowly build up to 30 seconds as you get fitter.

Swimming: Start by swimming as fast as you can for 25 meters in around 20 seconds, gradually increasing your speed as you get fitter.

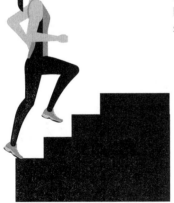

Stair climbing: Sprint hard up the stairs for 20 seconds, let your legs feel the burn, pause for 1–2 seconds, and then continue bounding for 20 seconds.

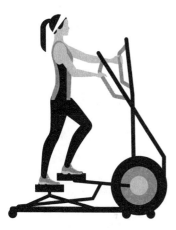

Cross-training: At the highest resistance, give a maximum effort for about 30 seconds before slowing down.

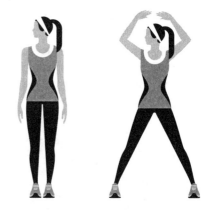

Jumping jacks: Do in a fast but controlled fashion for 30 seconds.

Jumping rope: Turn the rope as fast as you can—do as many rotations as you can within a minute.

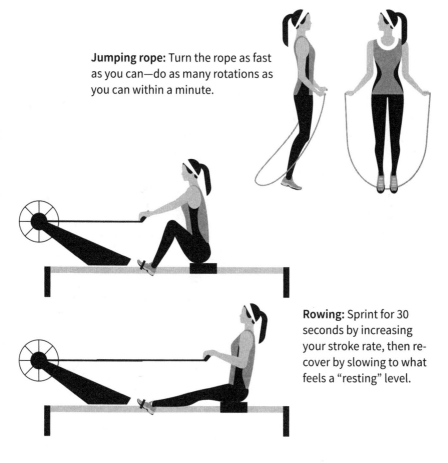

Rowing: Sprint for 30 seconds by increasing your stroke rate, then recover by slowing to what feels a "resting" level.

FastStrength

Depending on your fitness level, there are several workouts you can perform, all described on pages 312–326. Like FastFitness, these should be done 2–3 times a week, either in conjunction with FastFitness or alone. You can choose among the exercises below:

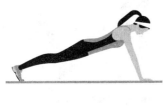

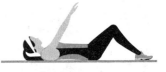

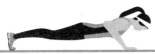

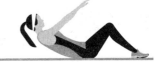

Push-ups: Do as many as you can in 30 seconds.

Abdominal crunches: Do as many as you can in 30 seconds in a fast but controlled manner.

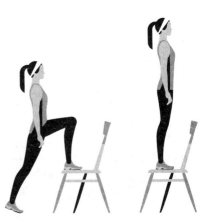

Wall sit: Hold this position for 30 seconds and rest 10 seconds between sets.

Step-ups on a chair: Perform with care but at a brisk pace for 30 seconds.

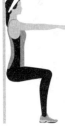

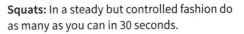

Squats: In a steady but controlled fashion do as many as you can in 30 seconds.

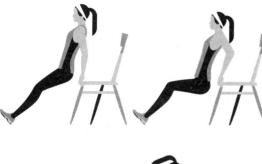

Tricep dips: Do as many as you can, quickly but controlled, for 30 seconds.

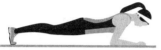

Plank: Hold this position as long as you can, and if you can't hold for 30 seconds, try 10 seconds, resting for 5 and holding for 10, for a total of 30 seconds.

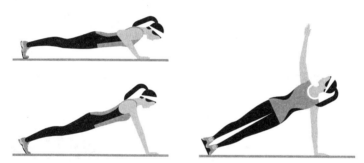

Push-up with rotation: In a controlled fashion, do as many as you can in 30 seconds.

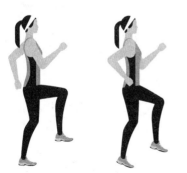

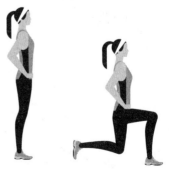

High-knee running: Do as many as you can in 30 seconds. You can start slowly, but ideally, these should be fast and high.

Lunges: In a steady but controlled manner, do as many as you can in 30 seconds.

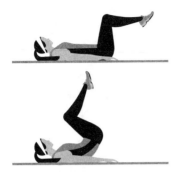
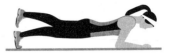
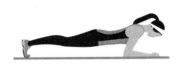

Reverse curl: Do as many as you can—slowly but controlled—in 30 seconds.

Plank with leg raise: Hold for as long as possible—ideally 30 seconds. If you can't, try holding for 10 seconds, resting for 5, holding for 10—for a total of 30 seconds.

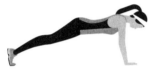
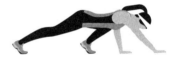

Bear crawl: Crawl for 10 seconds.

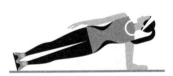

Side plank: Ideally hold for 30 seconds. If you can't, try holding for 10 seconds, resting for 5, holding for 10—for a total of 30 seconds.

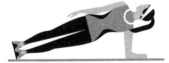
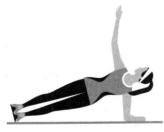
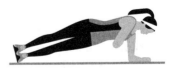

Side plank with reach around: In a steady but controlled fashion, do as many as you can in 30 seconds.

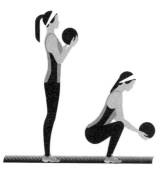

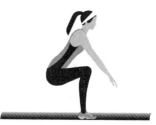

Log haul: Carry the rock, ball, or log a distance of 10 meters, aiming to move as quickly as possible.

Deep squat: Hold this position for 15 seconds.

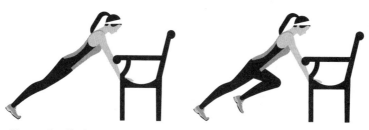

Mountain climber: In a controlled fashion, do as many as you can in 30 seconds.

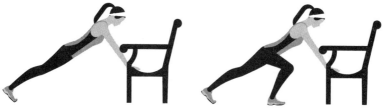

Squat thrust push-up: In a controlled fashion, do as many as you can in 30 seconds.

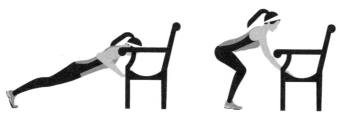

Bench get-up: In a controlled fashion, do as many as you can in 30 seconds.

Acknowledgments

This book would not have been possible without the many scientists who gave so generously of their time and research. They include Dr. Luigi Fontana of Washington University School of Medicine; Professor Mark Mattson of the National Institute on Aging; Dr. Krista Varady of the University of Illinois at Chicago; and Professor Valter Longo, director of the USC Longevity Institute.

A huge thanks to Aidan Laverty, editor of BBC's *Horizon*, who pointed me toward the brave new worlds of intermittent fasting and HIT, and to the entire production team, but especially Kate Dart and Roshan Samarasinghe. I'd also like to thank Janice Hadlow, who was brave enough to first put me in front of the camera and gave me the chance to try new things.

Thank you to Nicola Jeal at the *Times* for her constant ingenuity and support.

Acknowledgments

Our thanks also go to Rebecca Nicolson, Aurea Carpenter, and Emmie Francis at Short Books, for their hard work and immediate grasp of *The FastDiet*'s life-changing potential.

A big thanks to Toby MacDonald and Jenna Caldwell.

To Mimi, Aurea, and Rebecca for your friendship, editorial input, and unwavering support.

To Natalie, Andrew, Dan, and Sophie—for making it happen.

Also, many thanks to my general practitioner, Sally Jenkins, who has always responded with great good humor to my outlandish requests; it's not easy being doctor to a self-experimenter.

Michael Mosley
September 2015

Notes

Introduction to the FastDiet

1. Valter Longo and Mark Mattson, "Fasting: Molecular Mechanisms and Clinical Applications," *Cell Metabolism*, vol. 19, issue 2 (4 February 2014): 181–92.

Chapter One: The Science of Fasting

1. Barry M. Popkin and Kiyah J. Duffey, "Does hunger and satiety drive eating anymore? Increasing eating occasions and decreasing time between eating occasions in the United States," *American Journal of Clinical Nutrition* (May 2010).
2. Hana Kahleova, "Eating two larger meals a day (breakfast and lunch) is more effective than six smaller meals in a reduced-energy regimen for patients with type 2 diabetes: a randomized crossover study," *Diabetologia* (May 18, 2014), 57(8): 1552–60.
3. Mark Mattson and Edward Calabrese, "When a Little Poison is Good for You," *New Scientist* magazine (August 6, 2008): 36–39.
4. A. J. Carlson and F. Hoelzel, Department of Physiology, University of Chicago, "Apparent prolongation of the life span of rats by intermittent fasting," *Journal of Nutrition* (1945). http://jn.nutrition.org/content/31/3/363.full.pdf.
5. (http://www.nature.com/news/medical-research-treat-aging-1.15585)

Luigi Fontana et al., "Medical Research: Treat Aging," *Nature* (23 July 2014).

6. E. Bergamini, G. Cavallini, A. Donati, Z. Gori, "The role of autophagy in aging: its essential part in the anti-aging mechanism of caloric restriction," *Annals of the New York Academy of Science* (October 2007): 69–74.

7. Valter D. Longo, et al., "Prolonged Fasting Reduces IGF-1/PKA to Promote Hematopoietic-Stem-Cell-Based Regeneration and Reverse Immunosuppression," *Cell Stem Cell*; vol. 14, issue 6 (June 5, 2014): 810–23.

8. K. A. Varady, S. Bhutani, E. C. Church, M. Kempel, "Short-term modified alternate-day fasting: a novel dietary strategy for weight loss and cardio-protection in obese adults," *American Journal of Clinical Nutrition* (November 2009): 1138–43.

9. M. N. Harvie, "The effect of intermittent energy and carbohydrate restriction v. daily energy restriction on weight loss and metabolic disease risk markers in overweight women," *British Journal of Nutrition* (October 2103); 110 (8): 1534–47.

10. N. M. Hussin, S. Shahar, N. I. M. F. Teng, et al., "Efficacy of Fasting and Calorie Restriction (FCR) on Mood and Depression Among Aging Men," *The Journal of Nutrition, Health & Aging*, vol. 17, issue 8 (October 2013): 674–80.

11. M. Hatori, C. Vollmers, A. Zarrinpar, L. DiTacchio, et al., "Time-Restricted Feeding Without Reducing Caloric Intake Prevents Metabolic Diseases in Mice Fed a High-Fat Diet," *Cell Metabolism* (2012): 848–60.

12. K. I. Erickson, M. W. Voss, et al., Salk Institute, San Diego, CA, "Exercise training increases size of hippocampus and improves memory," *Proceedings of the National Academy of Science USA* (January 2011): 3017–22.

13. V. K. Halagappa, Z. Guo, M. Pearson, Y. Matsuoka, R. G. Cutler, F. M. Laferla, M. P. Mattson. National Institute on Aging, Baltimore, MD, "Intermittent fasting and caloric restriction ameliorate age-related behavioral deficits in the triple-transgenic mouse model of Alzheimer's disease," *Neurobiology of Disease* (April 2007): 212–20.

14. Y. Shirayama, A. C. Chen, S. Nakagawa, D. S. Russell, R. S. Duman, Yale University School of Medicine, New Haven, CT, "Brain-derived neurotrophic factor produces anti-depressant effects in behavioral models of depression," *Journal of Neuroscience* (April 2002): 3251–61.

15. K. Suemaru, Y. Kitamura, R. Cui, Y. Gomita, H. Araki. Department of
Clinical Pharmacology and Pharmacy, Brain Science, Ehime University Hospital, Japan, "Strategy to develop a new drug for treatment-resistant depression—role of electroconvulsive stimuli and BDNF,"
Yakugaku Zasshi (April 2007): 735–42.
16. N. Halberg, M. Henriksen, N. Söderhamn, B. Stallknecht, T. Ploug,
P. Schjerling, and F. Dela, Department of Muscle Research Centre,
The Panum Institute, University of Copenhagen, Denmark, "Effect of
intermittent fasting and refeeding on insulin action in healthy men,"
Journal of Applied Physiology (December 2005): 2128–36.
17. L. Raffaghello, C. Lee, F. M. Safdie, M. Wei, F. Madia, G. Bianchi,
V. D. Longo, Andrus Gerontology Center, Department of Biological
Sciences and Norris Cancer Center, University of Southern California, LA, CA, "Starvation-dependent differential stress resistance protects normal but not cancer cells against high-dose chemotherapy,"
*Proceedings of the National Academy of Sciences of the United States of
America* (June 2008): 8215–20.
18. C. Lee, V. Longo, et al., University of Southern California, "Fasting
Cycles Retard Growth of Tumors and Sensitize a Range of Cancer
Cell Types to Chemotherapy," *Science Translational Medicine* (February
2012).
19. F. M. Safdie, T. Dorff, V. Longo, et al., University of Southern California, "Fasting and Cancer Treatment in Humans," *Aging* 1, no. 12
(December 31, 2009): 988–1007.
20. James B. Johnson, et al., "Alternate Day Calorie Restriction Improves
Clinical Findings and Reduces Markers of Oxidative Stress and
Inflammation in Overweight Adults with Moderate Asthma Free,"
Radical Biology and Medicine Free (March 1, 2007): 42(5): 665–674.
21. M. Wolters, "Diet and psoriasis: experimental data and clinical evidence," *British Journal of Dermatology* (October 2005): 153(4): 706–14.
22. J. R. Stradling, J. H. Crosby, Osler Chest Unit, Churchill Hospital
Oxford, "Predictors and prevalence of obstructive sleep apnea and
snoring in 1001 middle aged men," *Thorax*, 46, no. 2 (February
1991): 85–90.

Chapter Two: The FastDiet in Practice

1. M. N. Harvie, et al., Genesis Prevention Centre, University Hospital
of South Manchester NHS Foundation Trust, UK, "The effects of

intermittent or continuous energy restriction on weight loss and metabolic disease risk markers: a randomized trial in young overweight women," *International Journal of Obesity* (London: May 2011): 714–27.

2. H. J. Leidy, M. Tang, C. Armstrong, C. B. Martin, W. W. Campbell, University of Missouri, "The Effects of Consuming Frequent, Higher Protein Meals on Appetite and Satiety During Weight Loss in Overweight/Obese Men," *Obesity* 19, no. 4 (2011): 818–24.

   A. Astrup, Department of Human Nutrition, Centre for Advanced Food Studies, Royal Veterinary & Agricultural University, Copenhagen, Denmark, "The satiating power of protein—a key to obesity prevention?" *American Society for Clinical Nutrition*, (July 2005): 1–2.

   T. Halton and F. Hu, Department of Nutrition, Harvard School of Public Health, Boston, MA, "The Effects of High Protein Diets on Thermogenesis, Satiety, and Weight Loss," *Journal of the American College of Nutrition* (October 2004): 37–85.

3. Valter D. Longo, et al., "Low Protein Intake Is Associated with a Major Reduction in IGF-1, Cancer, and Overall Mortality," *Cell Metabolism*, vol. 19, issue 3 (March 3, 2014): 407–417.

4. C. O'Neil and T. Nicklas, Louisiana State University Agricultural Center, Baton Rouge, LA, "Nut Consumption Is Associated with Decreased Health Risk Factors for Cardiovascular Disease and Metabolic Syndrome in US Adults," *Journal of the American College of Nutrition* (December 2011): 502–10.

   E. Ros, L. C. Tapsel, J. Sabate, Lipid Clinic, Endocrinology and Nutrition Service, Institut d'Investigacions Biomèdiques August Pi i Sunyer, Hospital Clínic, Barcelona, Spain, "Nuts and berries for heart health," *Current Atherosclerosis Reports* (November 2010): 397–406.

5. N. Dhurandhar, Pennington Biomedical Research Center, Louisiana, "Egg Proteins for Breakfast Keeps You Feeling Full for Longer."

6. Brian Wansink, *Mindless Eating—Why We Eat More Than We Think* (New York: Bantam-Dell, 2006).

7. T. Mann, A. J. Tomiyama, E. Westling, A. Lew, B. Samuels, J. Chatman, UCLA, "Medicare's search for effective obesity treatments: Diets are not the answer," *American Psychologist* (April 2007): 220–33.

8. Brian Wansink and Jeffrey Sobal, "Mindless Eating: The 200 Daily Food Decisions We Overlook," *Environment and Behavior* (January 2007).

Notes

9. B. Wansink, J. E. Painter, Y. K. Lee, "The Office Candy Dish: Proximity's Influence on Estimated and Actual Consumption," *International Journal of Obesity* (May 2006).

10. www.marksdailyapple.com/health-benefits-of-intermittentfasting/#axzz2DQjnYyUz.

11. K. Van Proeyen, K. Szlufcik, H. Nielens, K. Pelgrim, L. Deldicque, M. Hesselink, P. P. Van Veldhoven, P. Hespel, Research Centre for Exercise and Health, Department of Biomedical Kinesiology, Leuven, Belgium, "Training in the fasted state improves glucose tolerance during fat-rich diet," *Journal of Physiology* (November 2010): 4289–302.

12. Jack F. Hollis, et al., Kaiser Permanente's Center for Health Research, "Weight Loss During the Intensive Intervention Phase of the Weight-Loss Maintenance Trial," *American Journal of Preventive Medicine* (August 2008).

13. C. K. Morewedge, Y. E. Huh, and J. Vosgerau, Carnegie Mellon University, Pittsburgh, PA, "Thought for Food: Imagined Consumption Reduces Actual Consumption," *Science* (December 2010): 1530–3.

14. A. Fishbach, T. Eyal, S. R. Finkelstein, "How Positive and Negative Feedback Motivate Goal Pursuit," *Social and Personality Psychology Compass* (2010).

15. C. Zauner, B. Schneeweiss, A. Kranz, C. Madl, K. Ratheiser, L. Kramer, E. Roth, B. Schneider, and K. Lenz, University of Vienna, "Resting energy expenditure in short-term starvation," *American Journal of Nutrition* (June 2000).

16. M. W. Huff, Robarts Research Institute at the University of Western Ontario, Canada. "Nobiletin Attenuates VLDL Overproduction, Dyslipidemia, and Atherosclerosis in Mice With Diet-Induced Insulin Resistance," *American Journal of Diabetes* (May 2011).

17. E. E. Mulvihill, E. M. Alister, B. G. Sutherland, D. E. Telford, C. G. Sawyer, J. Y. Edwards, J. M. Markl, R. A. Hegele, M. W. Huff, Robarts Research Institute at the University of Western Ontario, Canada, "Naringenin prevents dyslipidemia, apolipoprotein B overproduction and hyperinsulinemia in LDL-receptor null mice with diet-induced insulin resistance," *Diabetes* (2009): 2198–210.

18. K. Fujioka, F. Greenway, J. Sheard, Y. Ying, Scripps Clinic, La Jolla, CA, "The effects of grapefruit on weight and insulin resistance: relationship to the metabolic syndrome," *Journal of Medicinal Food* (2006): 49–54.

19. D. Schrenk, Geisenheim Research Center, Germany, "Pectin, Fat Absorption, and Anti-Carcinogenic Effects," *Nutrition* (April 2008).

20. A. V. Rao; S. Agarwal, Department of Nutritional Sciences, Faculty of Medicine, University of Toronto, Canada, "Role of Antioxidant Lycopene in Cancer and Heart Disease," *Journal of the American College of Nutrition* (October 2000): 563–69.

21. J. Karppi, J. A. Laukkanen, J. Sivenius; K. Ronkainen, S. Kurl, Department of Medicine, Institute of Public Health and Clinical Nutrition, University of Eastern Finland, Kuopio, "Serum lycopene decreases the risk of stroke in men," *Neurology* 79, no. 15 (October 2012): 1540–47.

22. S. Moghe. Texas Woman's University, Denton, Texas, US, "Blueberries may inhibit development of fat cells," Federation of American Societies for Experimental Biology, *Science Daily* (April 2011).

23. B. Rolls, J. Flood, Penn State University, "Eating Soup Will Help Cut Calories at Meals," presented at the Experimental Biology Conference in Washington, DC (April 2007).

24. R. H. Liu, Department of Food Science, Cornell University, New York, "Thermal Processing Enhances the Nutritional Value of Tomatoes by Increasing Total Antioxidant Activity," *Journal of Agricultural and Food Chemistry* (April 2002).

25. C. Miglio, E. Chiavaro, A. Visconti, V. Foglian, Department of Public Health, University of Parma, Italy, "Effects of Different Cooking Methods on Nutritional and Physicochemical Characteristics of Selected Vegetables," *Journal of Agricultural and Food Chemistry* (December 2007): 139–47.

26. C. P. Herman and D. Mack, "Restrained and unrestrained eating," *Journal of Personality* 43, no. 1 (1975): 647–60.

27. E. J. Dhurandhar, J. Dawson, A. Alcorn, L. H. Larsen, E. Thomas, M. Cardel, A. Courland, A. Astrup, M. P. St. Onge, J. Hill, C. Apovian, J. Shikany, and D. Allison, "The effectiveness of breakfast recommendations on weight loss: a randomized controlled trial," *American Journal of Clinical Nutrition* (June 2014).

28. S. E. Swithers and T. L. Davidson, "Pavlovian Approach to the Problem of Obesity," Purdue University, IN, *International Journal of Obesity* (June 2004).

    S. E. Swithers and T. L. Davidson, "A Role for Sweet Taste: Calorie Predictive Relations in Energy Regulation by Rats," Purdue University, *Behavioral Neuroscience* (February 2008).

29. A. E. Mesas, L. M. Leon-Munoz, E. Lopez-Garcia, Department of Preventive Medicine and Public Health, School of Medicine, Universidad Autónoma de Madrid, Spain, "The effect of coffee on blood pressure and cardiovascular disease in hypertensive individuals," *American Journal of Clinical Nutrition* (2011): 1113–26.

S. Larsson and N. Orsini, National Institute of Environmental Medicine, Karolinska Institutet, Stockholm, Sweden, "Coffee Consumption and Risk of Stroke: A Dose-Response Meta-Analysis of Prospective Studies," *American Journal of Epidemiology* (September 2011): 993–1001.

Anna Floegel, Tobias Pischon, Manuela M. Bergmann, Birgit Teucher, Rudolf Kaaks, Heiner Boeing, European Prospective Investigation into Cancer and Nutrition (EPIC), Germany, "Coffee consumption and risk of chronic disease," *American Society for Nutrition* (April 2012): 901–8.

30. D. T. Kirkendall, J. B. Leiper, Z. Bartagi, J. Dvorak, Y. Zerguini, FIFA Medical Assessment and Research Centre, Schulthess Clinic, Zurich, Switzerland, "The influence of Ramadan on physical performance measures in young Muslim footballers," *Journal of Sports Science* 26, supplement 3 (December 2008): S15–27.

31. K. Van Proeyen, et al., Research Centre for Exercise and Health, Department of Biomedical Kinesiology, Leuven, Belgium, "Beneficial Metabolic Adaptations due to Endurance Exercise Training in the Fasted State," *Journal of Applied Physiology*, 110, no. 1 (January 2011): 236–45.

32. M. P. Harber, A. R. Konopka, B. Jemiolo, S. W. Trappe, T. A. Trappe, P. T. Reidy, Human Performance Laboratory, Ball State University, Muncie, IN, "Muscle protein synthesis and gene expression during recovery from aerobic exercise in the fasted and fed states," *American Journal of Physiology*, 299, no. 5 (November 2010): R1254–62.

33. L. Deldicque, K. De Bock, M. Maris, M. Ramaekers, H. Nielens, M. Francaux, P. Hespel, Department of Biomedical Kinesiology, Leuven, Belgium, "Increased p70s6k phosphorylation during intake of a protein-carbohydrate drink following resistance exercise in the fasted state," *European Journal of Applied Physiology* (March 2010).

34. K. Van Proeyen, K. Szlufcik, H. Nielens, K. Pelgrim, L. Deldicque, M. Hesselink, P. P. Van Veldhoven, P. Hespel, Research Centre for Exercise and Health, Department of Biomedical Kinesiology, Leuven, Belgium, "Training in the fasted state improves glucose tolerance during fat-rich diet," *Journal of Physiology* (November 2010).

35. G. Reynolds, "Phys Ed: The Benefits of Exercising Before Breakfast," *New York Times*, December 15, 2010. http://well.blogs.nytimes.com /2010/12/15/phys-ed-the-benefits-ofexercising-before-breakfast /?src=me&ref=general.

36. M. A. Tarnopolsky, McMaster University Medical Center, Hamilton, Ontario, Canada, "Gender Differences in Substrate Metabolism During Endurance Exercise," *Canadian Journal of Applied Physiology*, 25, no. 4 (2000): 312–27.

37. S. R. Stannard, A. J. Buckley, J. A. Edge, M. W. Thompson, Institute of Food Nutrition and Human Health, Massey University, New Zealand, "Adaptations to skeletal muscle with endurance exercise training in the acutely fed versus overnight-fasted state," *Journal of Science and Medicine in Sport*, 13, no. 4 (July 2010): 465–69.

Chapter Four: The Truth About Exercise

1. James Woodcock, et al., "Non-vigorous physical activity and all-cause mortality: systematic review and meta-analysis of cohort studies." *International Journal of Epidemiology* 40, no. 1 (2011): 121–38.

2. David Spiegelhalter, "Using speed of ageing and "microlives" to communicate the effects of lifetime habits and environment." *BMJ* 345 (2012), doi: http://dx.doi.org/10.1136/bmj.e8223.

3. Stanley J. Colcombe, et al., "Aerobic Exercise Training Increases Brain Volume in Aging Humans." *Journal of Gerontology: Medical Sciences* 61A, no. 11 (2006): 1166–1170.

4. Laura DeFina et al., "The Association Between Midlife Cardiorespiratory Fitness Levels and Later-Life Dementia: A Cohort Study."*Annals of Internal Medicine* 158, no. 3 (2013): 162–168. doi:10.7326/0003-4819-158-3-201302050-00005.

5. Hélène Sandmark, "Musculoskeletal dysfunction in physical education teachers." *Occupational and Environmental Medicine* 57, no. 10 (2000): 673–677, doi: 10.1136/oem.57.10.673.

6. James H. O'Keefe and Carl J. Lavie, "Run for your life . . . at a comfortable speed and not too far." *Heart* (2012), doi:10.1136/heartjnl-2012-302886.

7. Peter Schnohr et al., "Longevity in Male and Female Joggers: the Copenhagen City Heart Study." *American Journal of Epidemiology* 177:7 (2013): 683–9, doi:10.1093/aje/kws301.

8. Raymond Noordam, et al., "High serum glucose levels are associated

with a higher perceived age." *Age: Journal of the American Aging Association* 35, no. 1 (2011): 189–95.

9. Mehrdad Heydari, Judith Freund, and Stephen H. Boutcher, "The Effect of High-Intensity Intermittent Exercise on Body Composition of Overweight Young Males," *Journal of Obesity* 2012 (2012): doi:10.1155/2012/480467.

10. John M. Jakicic, et al., "Effect of exercise on 24-month weight loss maintenance in overweight women." *Archives of Internal Medicine* 168, no. 14 (2008): 1550–9.

11. Adapted from Cameron Hall et al., "Energy expenditure of walking and running: comparison with prediction equations." *Medicine & Science in Sports & Exercise* 36, no. 12 (2004): 2128–34.

12. E. G. Trapp et al., "The effects of high-intensity intermittent exercise training on fat loss and fasting insulin levels of young women." *International Journal of Obesity* 32, no. 4 (2008): 684–91, doi:10.1038/sj.ijo.0803781.

13. D. M. Thomas et al., "Why do individuals not lose more weight from an exercise intervention at a defined dose? An energy balance analysis." *Obesity Reviews* 13, no. 10 (2012): 835–847.

14. C. D. Lee et al., "US weight guidelines: is it also important to consider cardiorespiratory fitness?" *International Journal of Obesity and Related Metabolic Disorders* 22, sup. 2 (1998): S2–7.

15. Surabhi Bhutani et al., "Alternate day fasting and endurance exercise combine to reduce body weight and favorably alter plasma lipids in obese humans." *Obesity* 21, no. 7 (2013): 1370–9.

Chapter Five: What Is FastExercise?

1. Herman Pontzer et al., "Hunter-Gatherer Energetics and Human Obesity." *PLoS ONE* 7, no. 7 (2012): doi:10.1371/journal.pone.0040503.

2. James H. O'Keefe et al., "Achieving Hunter-gatherer Fitness in the 21st Century: Back to the Future." *The American Journal of Medicine* 123, no. 12 (2010): 1082–1086, doi:10.1016/j.amjmed.2010.04.026.

3. Burgomaster, Kirsten A., et al. "Six sessions of sprint interval training increases muscle oxidative potential and cycle endurance capacity in humans." *Journal of Applied Physiology* 98, no. 6 (2005) 1985–1990, doi:10.1152/japplphysiol.01095.2004.

4. Martin J. Gibala et al., "Short-term sprint interval *versus* traditional endurance training: similar initial adaptations in human skeletal

muscle and exercise performance." September 15, 2006 575, no. 3 (2006): 901–911, doi:10.1113/jphysiol.2006.112094.

5. Martin J. Gibala et al., "Physiological adaptations to low-volume, high-intensity interval training in health and disease." *The Journal of Physiology* 590, no. 5 (2012): 1077–1084, doi:10.1113/jphysiol.2011.224725.

6. E. G. Trapp et al., "The effects of high-intensity intermittent exercise training on fat loss and fasting insulin levels of young women." *International Journal of Obesity* 32, no. 4 (2008): 684–91, doi:10.1038/sj.ijo.0803781.

7. Mehrdad Heydari, Judith Freund, and Stephen H. Boutcher, "The Effect of High-Intensity Intermittent Exercise on Body Composition of Overweight Young Males," *Journal of Obesity* 2012 (2012): doi:10.1155/2012/480467.

8. Rebecca E. K. Macpherson et al., "Run Sprint Interval Training Improves Aerobic Performance but Not Maximal Cardiac Output." *Medicine & Science in Sports & Exercise* 43, no. 1 (2011): 115–122, doi:10.1249/MSS.0b013e3181e5eacd.

9. David Thivel et al., "The 24-h Energy Intake of Obese Adolescents Is Spontaneously Reduced after Intensive Exercise: A Randomized Controlled Trial in Calorimetric Chambers." *PLoS ONE* 7, no. 1 (2012), doi:10.1371/journal.pone.0029840.

10. Aaron Y. Sim et al., "High-intensity intermittent exercise attenuates ad-libitum energy intake." *International Journal of Obesity* (2013): doi:10.1038/ijo.2013.102.

11. Laura Karavita et al., "Individual responses to combined endurance and strength training in older adults." *Medicine & Science in Sports & Exercise* 43, no. 3 (2011): 484–90, doi:10.1249/MSS.0b013e3181f1bf0d.

12. Christian M. O'Connor et al., "Efficacy and Safety of Exercise Training in Patients With Chronic Heart Failure: HF-ACTION Randomized Controlled Trial." *JAMA* 301, no. 14 (2009): 1439–1450, doi:10.1001/jama.2009.454.

13. Øivind Rognmo et al., "Cardiovascular Risk of High- Versus Moderate-Intensity Aerobic Exercise in Coronary Heart Disease Patients." *Circulation* 126, no. 12 (2012): 1436–40, doi:10.1161/CIRCULATIONAHA.112.123117.

14. Philippe Meyer et al., "High-Intensity Aerobic Interval Exercise in Chronic Heart Failure." *Current Heart Failure Reports* 10, no. 2 (2013): 130–138, doi:10.1007/s11897-013-0130-3.

Chapter Six: FastExercise: The Workouts

1. Shrier, Ian. "When and Whom to Stretch? Gauging the Benefits and Drawbacks for Individual Patients." *The Physician and Sportsmedicine Journal* 33, no. 3 (2005): 22–6, doi:10.3810/psm.2005.03.61.

2. Erik Witvrouw et al., "Stretching and injury prevention: an obscure relationship." *Sports Medicine* 34, no. 7 (2004):443–9, doi:10.2165 /00007256-200434070-00003.

3. Roberta Y. W. Law and Robert D. Herbert, "Warm-up reduces delayed-onset muscle soreness but cooldown does not: a randomized controled trial." *Australian Journal of Physiotherapy*, 53, no. 2 (2007): 91–95, doi: http://dx.doi.org/10.1016/S0004-9514(07)70041-7.

4. Richard S. Metcalfe, et al., "Towards the minimal amount of exercise for improving metabolic health: beneficial effects of reduced-exertion high-intensity interval training." *European Journal of Applied Physiology* 112, no. 7 (2012): 2767–75, doi:10.1007/s00421-011-2254-z.

5. Kristen A. Burgomaster et al., "Similar metabolic adaptations during exercise after low volume sprint interval and traditional endurance training in humans." *Journal of Physiology* 586, no. 1 (2008): 151–60.

6. E. G. Trapp et al., "The effects of high-intensity intermittent exercise training on fat loss and fasting insulin levels of young women." *International Journal of Obesity* 32, no. 4 (2008): 684–91, doi:10.1038 /sj.ijo.0803781.

7. Arnt Erik Tjønna et al., "Low- and high-volume of intensive endurance training significantly improves maximal oxygen uptake after 10-weeks of training in healthy men." *PLoS ONE* 8, no. 5 (2013), doi:10.1371/journal.pone.0065382.

8. Brett Klika and Chris Jordan, "High-intensity circuit training using body weight: maximum results with minimal investment." *ACSM's Health & Fitness Journal* 17, no. 3 (2013): 8–13, doi:10.1249/ FIT.0b013e31828cb1e8.

Chapter Seven: FastExercise in Practice

1. Maria Maraki et al., "Acute effects of a single exercise class on appetite, energy intake and mood. Is there a time of day effect?" *Appetite* 45 (2005): 272–278, doi:10.1016/j.appet.2005.07.005.

2. Sedliak, Milan, et al. "Effect of Time-of-Day-Specific Strength Training on Serum Hormone Concentrations and Isometric Strength in Men." *Chronobiology International* 24, no. 6 (2007): 1159–1177, doi:10.1080/07420520701800686.

3. Christopher D. Black et al., "Ginger (Zingiber officinale) Reduces Muscle Pain Caused by Eccentric Exercise." *The Journal of Pain* 11, no. 9 (2010): 894–903, doi: http://dx.doi.org/10.1016/j.jpain.2009.12.013.

Chapter Eight: Michael's Guide to Keeping Active

1. David W. Dunstan et al., "Breaking up prolonged sitting reduces postprandial glucose and insulin responses." *Diabetes Care* 35, no. 5 (2012): 976–83, doi: 10.2337/dc11-1931.

2. James O. Hill et al., *The Step Diet: Count Steps, Not Calories to Lose Weight and Keep It Off Forever.* (New York: Workman Publishing Company, 2004).

3. Kristian Karstoft et al., "The Effects of Free-Living Interval-Walking Training on Glycemic Control, Body Composition, and Physical Fitness in Type 2 Diabetic Patients: A randomized, controlled trial." *Diabetes Care* 36 (2013): 228–236, doi:10.2337/dc12-0658.

4. Ken-Ichi Nemoto et al., "Effects of High-Intensity Interval Walking Training on Physical Fitness and Blood Pressure in Middle-Aged and Older People," *Mayo Clinic Proceedings* 82, no. 7 (2007): 803–811, doi: http://dx.doi.org/10.4065/82.7.803.

Index

A

abdominal crunches, 315, 378
activity, 110, 223, 355
   calories burned doing
      different activities, 371–75
   heart failure and, 284
   hunter-gatherers and,
      248–52, 355
   Michael's guide to keeping
      active, 343–54
   sendentariness and, 344–48,
      356–57
   stairs and, 348–49
   12 easy ways to introduce,
      352–54
   walking, *see* walking
   see also exercise
adenosine triphosphate (ATP),
   260
adrenaline, 265–66
aerobic exercise, 262
aerobic fitness, 231, 276
   assessing, 363–64
Aerobics (Cooper), 367
alcohol, 124
alternate-day fasting (ADF),
   32–35, 59, 138

asthma and, 56–57
   exercise and, 110, 244
aging, 21, 23, 141
Allen, Woody, 39
Alzheimer's disease, 40, 41, 42,
   45
*American College of Sports
   Medicine's Health & Fitness
   Journal*, 313, 326
American Diabetes Association,
   114
American Journal of Medicine, 250
American Lung Association, 297
anatomy changes, 91
Anderson, Tracey, 247
anthocyanins, 339
antioxidants, 19, 224
appetite, 14, 101, 119
   changes in, 92
   exercise and, 266
   HIT and, 266, 268–73
   see also hunger
Appetite, 330
Armstrong, Neil, 217
arthritis, 228
aspirin, 292
asthma, 55–57

Index

About the Authors

Michael Mosley did a first degree at Oxford University before training to be a doctor at the Royal Free Hospital in London. After qualifying he joined the BBC, where he has been a science journalist, an executive producer, and more recently, a well-known television presenter. He has written and presented series on BBC One, Two, Three, and Four as well as BBC Radio Four; and has won numerous television awards, including a Royal Television Society award, and been named Medical Journalist of the Year by the British Medical Association. He is married to a doctor and has four children.

Mimi Spencer is a feature writer, columnist, and the author of *101 Things to Do Before You Diet*.

Peta Bee is an award-winning journalist who writes regularly for the *Times*, *Daily Mail*, and *Sunday Times*. She has degrees in sports science and nutrition and is a qualified running coach. Peta won the Medical Journalists' Association's Freelance Journalist of the Year award in 2008 and 2012 and appears regularly on television and radio. She has published several books on health and fitness and lives with her family in Berkshire, England.